T0245215

The Associate Professor Guidebook

Laura Weiss Roberts
Editor

The Associate Professor Guidebook

Continuing the Journey to Professor

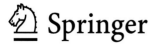 Springer

Editor
Laura Weiss Roberts, MD, MA
Chairman and Katharine Dexter McCormick
  and Stanley McCormick Memorial Professor
Department of Psychiatry and Behavioral Sciences
Stanford University
Stanford, CA, USA

ISBN 978-3-319-28000-4   ISBN 978-3-319-28001-1 (eBook)
DOI 10.1007/978-3-319-28001-1

Library of Congress Control Number: 2016932387

Springer Cham Heidelberg New York Dordrecht London

Printed on acid-free paper

Springer International Publishing AG Switzerland is part of Springer Science+Business Media (www.springer.com)

For our sweet Tuli

Preface

Many academic faculty members get stuck at the associate professor level. They are meritorious. They have been recognized for their great promise and clear contributions to their institutions by being promoted from the assistant professor rank. They are important to their colleagues and their students and their organization's leaders. And they together represent the cadre of future leaders of academic medicine. And yet, somehow, they get stuck.

Some associate professors stay in academia, fulfilling the same duties that they did as assistant professors and feeling uncertain about where they "fit" on their faculty. Many remain in academia, shouldering more and more responsibilities for their institution, but not able to advance their scholarship or build their national reputations in order to attain promotion to professor rank. Some cannot imagine taking on, or being chosen for, leadership roles at their institutions. Some move to roles outside of academia, entering private or group practice or industry roles, where they can no longer mentor, teach, or pursue scholarship but perhaps enjoy a better paycheck. On the professional developmental career path, the associate professor often walks the longest mile.

Academic mentorship tends to focus on early career faculty, helping instructors or assistant professors get (and keep) their jobs and explaining the mysteries of the academy. For associate professors, they often understand too well the pressures and politics of the academy—and yet they may not see how they can "break through" to more senior leadership roles, contributing to their fields on a national level and entering into more influential roles at their institutions. The *Associate Professor Guidebook*, derived from a broader text *The Academic Medicine Handbook*, has been created specifically to address these challenges that academic faculty members encounter and are often felt most keenly by associate professors, in advancing their careers and feeling fulfilled along the way.

The *Associate Professor Guidebook* has 22 chapters that seek to enhance strengths of particular value to academic faculty at the associate professor level. Some of these strengths relate to fostering and sustaining one's sense of well-being in academic settings. Examples include how to manage time, how to cultivate a healthy life balance, how to manage personal finances, and how to put together a promotion package and create an effective narrative for traditional and nontraditional academic careers. Other strengths emphasized in this guidebook relate to developing capacities that are helpful in serving academic institutions at a higher level, setting the stage for future leadership roles as a professor. Examples include how to be a good mentor, how to lead committees, how to build a national reputation, how to collaborate interprofessionally, how to understand budgets, how to engage in strategic planning, and how to understand how money works in academic medicine. With emphasis on the cultivation of "soft" and "hard" skills, this guidebook is targeted to help associate professors prepare themselves for, and aspire to, more in their academic careers.

Associate professors are important to academic medicine. They are "keepers"—individuals recognized by their institutions for their great work and great promise and who have been promoted to the senior ranks of academic medicine. The continued career development of these individuals is so very crucial to their students, their colleagues, and their senior leaders. Even more, associate professors represent the living "succession plan" for academic medicine, which has been entrusted with creating a better future for humanity. This guidebook is intended to foster the strengths of my associate professor colleagues in recognition of their critically important roles, today and tomorrow, in academic medicine.

Stanford, CA, USA   Laura Weiss Roberts, MD, MA

Acknowledgments

I wish to express my gratitude to my dear colleagues who have contributed to this handbook as a gift to the future of academic medicine and a kindness to me personally.

Ann Tennier, editorial assistant-extraordinaire, has done (as always) superb work in advancing this project. For this, and many other reasons, she has my deepest thanks.

Contents

..

Contributors

Jerald Belitz, Ph.D. Department of Psychiatry, University of New Mexico, Albuquerque, NM, USA

Jonathan F. Borus, M.D. Department of Psychiatry, Brigham and Women's Hospital and Harvard Medical School, Boston, MA, USA

Linda M. Boxer, M.D., Ph.D. Department of Medicine, Stanford University, Stanford, CA, USA

Judith P. Cain Department of Medicine, Stanford University, Stanford, CA, USA

Diana Carmichael, M.H.A. AMC Strategies, LLC, Los Angeles, CA, USA

Margaret S. Chisolm, M.D. Department of Psychiatry and Behavioral Sciences, Johns Hopkins University, Baltimore, MD, USA

Marcia J. Cohen, M.B.A. Stanford University School of Medicine, Stanford, CA, USA

Ann Freeman Cook, M.P.A., B.A., Ph.D. Department of Psychology, The University of Montana, Missoula, MT, USA

Arthur R. Derse, M.D., J.D. Center for Bioethics and Medical Humanities, Medical College of Wisconsin, Milwaukee, WI, USA

Laura B. Dunn, M.D. Department of Psychiatry, University of California, San Francisco, San Francisco, CA, USA

Sabine C. Girod, M.D., D.D.S., Ph.D., F.A.C.S. Department of Surgery (Oral Medicine & Maxillofacial Surgery), Stanford School of Medicine, Stanford, CA, USA

Daisy Grewal, Ph.D. Department of Office of Diversity and Leadership, Stanford School of Medicine, Stanford, CA, USA

Christopher Guest, M.D., Ph.D. Department of Emergency Medicine, Stanford University Hospital, Stanford, CA, USA

Nathan Hantke, M.S. Department of Clinical Psychology, Marquette University, Milwaukee, WI, USA

Helena Hoas, Ph.D. Department of Psychology, University of Montana, Missoula, MT, USA

Robert K. Jackler, M.D. Department of Otolaryngology—Head and Neck Surgery, Stanford University Medical Center, Stanford, CA, USA

Michael D. Jibson, M.D., Ph.D. Department of Psychiatry, University of Michigan Health System, Ann Arbor, MI, USA

Edward Kass, Ph.D. Department of Organization, Leadership, and Communication, University of San Francisco, School of Management, San Francisco, CA, USA

Jennifer R. Kogan, M.D. Department of Medicine, Perelman School of Medicine at the University of Pennsylvania, Philadelphia, PA, USA

Manwai Candy Ku, Ph.D. Department of Office of Diversity and Leadership, Stanford University School of Medicine, Stanford, CA, USA

Teresita McCarty, M.D. Assessment and Learning, University of New Mexico, Albuquerque, NM, USA

Cynthiane Morgenweck, M.D. Center for Bioethics and Medical Humanities, Medical College of Wisconsin, Milwaukee, WI, USA

Christine Moutier, M.D. Department of Psychiatry, University of California, San Diego, School of Medicine, La Jolla, CA, USA

David O'Brien, M.H.A. Office of Institutional Planning, Stanford University School of Medicine, Menlo Park, CA, USA

David J. Peterson, M.B.A., F.A.C.M.P.E. Department of Psychiatry and Behavioral Medicine, Medical College of Wisconsin, Milwaukee, WI, USA

Robert C. Robbins, M.D. Texas Medical Center, Houston, TX, USA

Laura Weiss Roberts, M.D., M.A. Department of Psychiatry and Behavioral Sciences, Stanford University, Stanford, CA, USA

Upinder Singh, M.D. Department of Medicine and Microbiology and Immunology, Stanford University, Stanford, CA, USA

Rebecca Smith-Coggins, M.D. Department of Emergency Medicine, Stanford University Medical Center, Stanford, CA, USA

Ryan Spellecy, Ph.D. Center for Bioethics and Medical Humanities, Medical College of Wisconsin, Milwaukee, WI, USA

David K. Stevenson, M.D. Department of Pediatrics, Stanford University School of Medicine, Stanford, CA, USA

Roger Strode, J.D., C.P.A. Department of Health Care, Foley & Lardner LLP, Chicago, IL, USA

Mickey Trockel, M.D., Ph.D. Department of Psychiatry and Behavioral Sciences, Stanford University, Stanford, CA, USA

Hannah Valantine, M.D. Department of Office of Diversity and Leadership/Cardiovascular Medicine, Stanford University School of Medicine, Stanford, CA, USA

Penelope Zeifert, Ph.D. Department of Neurology and Neurological Sciences, Stanford University Medical Center, Stanford, CA, USA

Sidney Zisook, M.D. Department of Psychiatry, University of California, San Francisco, San Francisco, CA, USA

Veterans Affairs San Diego Healthcare System and Veterans Medical and Research Foundation, La Jolla, CA, USA

How to Find Your Path in Academic Medicine

1

Laura Weiss Roberts

> *Although the world is full of suffering, it is full also of the overcoming of it.*
>
> Helen Keller

Academic medicine exists to create a better future for all of humanity. Medical school faculty fulfill this awesome responsibility through present-day effort in five interdependent realms: advancing science, engaging in clinical innovation and service, fostering multidisciplinary education, collaborating to address societal needs, and nurturing leadership and professionalism. Faculty investigators seek new knowledge to help understand the biological basis of health and disease as well as the psychological, cultural, and social determinants of illness. Academic clinicians apply scientific evidence to help individual patients, to establish better practices, and to create effective systems of care for entire populations. Teachers teach. Medical school educators impart knowledge, build competencies, and inspire students across the many disciplines of the health professions. Faculty work with diverse partners to define

L.W. Roberts, M.D., M.A. (✉)
Department of Psychiatry and Behavioral Sciences, Stanford University,
401 Quarry Road, Stanford, CA, USA
e-mail: RobertsL@stanford.edu

© Springer International Publishing Switzerland 2016   1
L.W. Roberts (ed.), *The Associate Professor Guidebook*,
DOI 10.1007/978-3-319-28001-1_1

and take on concerns affecting the health of communities, whether local or global. Medical school faculty, in turn, help cultivate the next generation of leaders—people who will be prepared to offer expertise and wise judgment in broad policy efforts, scientific inquiry, and organizational responses to issues of importance to human health. Through these efforts, individually and collectively, academic faculty members have stepped forward to address vast health problems that do and will affect all people. On the shoulders of academic medicine rides the hope that the world's next generation will live better lives and endure fewer burdens of suffering, disability, and premature mortality.

When entering the profession of academic medicine, it is clear that the path ahead will thus be one of great purpose and hard work. Harder to discern at the outset are three other aspects of a career in academic medicine that are immensely valued by experienced faculty. First, the work itself is creative and complex. Second, the colleagues are extraordinary. And, third, the environment of academic medicine continuously—perhaps relentlessly—causes faculty members to question, to learn, and to extend themselves. *Meaning, effort, creativity, colleagueship*, and *growth*. These elements define the experience of a life dedicated to academic medicine and, taken together, they give rise to careers of unimagined achievement and distinct worth for those who choose this path.

> *A hero is someone who understands the responsibility that comes with his freedom.*
>
> Bob Dylan

So, how does one choose the path of academic medicine? For some, the aspirational "calling" of helping humanity through discovery or healing will draw them to this field. For many, the love of teaching makes alternative careers—a future without connection to students each day—far less compelling. For others, academic medicine will provide the optimal, most exciting, or only settings for their scientific work. For some "bitten by the bug" of academic medicine, the opportunity to pursue the multiple missions of doing science, caring for patients, teaching, collaborating, and leading plaited as one cohesive endeavor will be irresistible.

And for yet others, entering academic medicine may simply feel intuitive and logical—encouraged by their mentors and surrounded by friends, moving from the role as student to faculty member in a familiar context becomes an obvious "next step" in their careers. Perhaps all of these influences have some part in the decisions of students to choose academic medicine.

Whatever the reasons, my sense is that nearly all early-career faculty members experience, as I did, an unsettling combination of feeling overly schooled and, yet, still underprepared. Decades of formal education, as it turns out, are insufficient for some of the unexpected and labor-intensive everyday duties of the instructor/assistant professor, such as writing letters of recommendation, sitting on committees or, worse, seeking committee approvals, formatting one's curriculum vitae, obtaining a "360" evaluation, undergoing compliance audits, fulfilling quality performance metrics, and the like. These tasks are not among those that an early academic thinks of when aspiring to better the human condition. Moreover, the dynamics among the faculty may be rather unexpected. Rather. The esteem, as well as the size of office or laboratory and financial compensation, accorded to an early-career faculty member may also seem just a bit thin after all the years of training. Managing these duties and dynamics and becoming a graceful self-advocate are, one quickly learns, essential to one's success in an academic career. Without some savvy in handling these "fundamentals" in the culture of medical schools, it will be difficult to turn to the bigger work of academic medicine.

Recognition of the importance of these basic, but typically untaught, skills for faculty members across academic medicine serves as the origin of this handbook. The text is organized into eight sections that encompass major domains, duties, and developmental aspects of faculty life. The sections are the following: approaching the profession of academic medicine, getting established, approaching work with colleagues, writing and evaluating manuscripts, conducting empirical research, developing administrative skills, advancing along academic paths, and ensuring personal well-being. Every section will be salient for all academic faculty members—the clinical educator should understand the process that translational scientist colleagues undergo in competing for research grants, for example, and the laboratory scientist should understand the nature of bedside teaching. Such understanding will foster collegiality and it will ensure greater fairness in accomplishing the many citizenship tasks of academic environments, such as when serving on a Promotion and Tenure (or "P & T") committee. The subjects of individual chapters are wide-ranging, derived from my own observations and impressions of what early career faculty "need to know" to navigate the course ahead. Examples of a chapter from each section include how to manage time effectively, how to give a lecture, how to approach the relationship with a mentor, how to write for publication, how to prepare a first grant application, how to negotiate, how to develop a national reputation, and how to manage personal finances. My hope in envisioning and assembling this handbook is that it will assist faculty to be effective and personally fulfilled as they progress through their careers in academic medicine.

Whatever you are, be a good one.

Abraham Lincoln

People who flourish in academic medicine possess certain qualities that allow them to adapt to the diverse and specific ecologies of medical school environments. Years ago Hilty and I observed that our most successful colleagues have several common attributes—beyond having a sense of purpose and the willingness to work hard, they are creative, organized, and tenacious; they foster good will; and they are open to opportunity [1]. As I have seen exceptional careers become damaged, and devastated, in my 19 years as an academic faculty member, I have come to understand that professional integrity, presupposed in the prior list, should be made explicit as a "necessary precondition" for effective academic careers. With experience in leadership roles, I also now include among the characteristics of the strongest faculty the ability to communicate the value of one's work to others and awareness of one's limitations and willingness to compensate, adapt, or reposition accordingly. Knowledge of the overall organization and governance of medical schools and understanding of how medical school realities are shaped by county, state, and federal resources, regulatory agencies, and public policy are also qualities that help faculty do well as they mature within the field. Dedication to the success of others within an academic organization (students, staff, peers, near-peers, or deans) and outside of the academic organization (affiliated institutions, community partners, professional colleagues, or governmental or nongovernmental entities) is another discernible quality of great academic faculty members. All of these characteristics allow a faculty member to thrive in medical school environments, advancing their careers but also supporting the value of these organizations in society.

Indeed, though they represent the "universe" for academic faculty, medical schools are relatively few in number and vary greatly. The Association of American Medical Colleges (AAMC, www.aamc.org) is an organization that represents all of the accredited medical schools in the USA and Canada, their major teaching hospitals and health systems, and key academic and scientific societies in the two countries. At the time of this writing, the AAMC has 137 medical schools in the USA and 17 in Canada, with eight more schools launched and moving toward accreditation by the Liaison Committee on Medical Education, a joint endeavor of the AAMC and the American Medical Association. The AAMC estimates that 128,000 faculty members, 75,000 medical students, and 110,000 resident physicians work within these academic medical organizations. Given that the population of the United States today is estimated to be 313.6 million people and of Canada is 33.5 million people, the number of medical schools is small by any count and the ratio of faculty-to-general population is strikingly low. Keeping the academic workforce robust, given its responsibilities to the many people it serves, is thus essential.

Medical schools must meet clear standards, but are quite different in their scope of activities, priorities, settings, finances, governance, and cultures. All provide high-quality education, though through remarkably diverse curricula. All must have teaching-related clinical services in general and specialty areas. Some medical schools have robust federal research funding for science, whereas others have nearly none. Some medical schools are financially sturdy while others find themselves frequently near fiscal collapse, trading program closure for the opportunity for the organization to survive another week. Some medical schools have as their primary task educating rural care providers to serve the health of neighboring communities, and some see their foremost duty as driving forward the most innovative basic and translational science that will transform all of our current understanding of human health and disease. Some medical schools ("medical colleges") are independent and free-standing, and others reside on a university campus embedded in a health sciences center with companion nursing, dental, and other health professional schools. Culturally, some medical schools take great pride in their elite standing while others, some of the best schools among them, have a much more down-to-earth nature.

Such diverse environments suggest the value of a diverse set of people suited to the work of academic medicine. Scientists, clinicians, teachers, leaders, and "mosaics" all belong. Success as a faculty member will thus involve looking for the "best fit" between the person and the organization and, more specifically, the person at a particular point in his or her professional development and the organization at a particular point in its history. Extraordinary ("top tier") institutions can help advance stellar careers through exceptional mentors and facilities, but for some early-career faculty it may be difficult to get the recognition and opportunities that they would receive as a "bigger fish" in a "smaller pond." More modest institutions may not have the resources to afford the larger commitments needed by their talented, let alone their "superstar," faculty, however. Institutional history is also relevant in that academic entities that have grown through investments in basic science or, alternatively, in clinical expansion are likely to adhere to their past successes in future decisions. Academic programs that have thrived by taking "high-risk, high-gain" commitments are likely to be bolder whereas fiscally strapped entities or those that have, let's say, just undergone investigation by the federal government for human subjects compliance concerns may be very conservative in their decision-making. These factors, though they seem far-removed from the everyday life of the individual faculty member, shape the milieu and can greatly influence the academic work that each person undertakes.

In thinking through whether a particular academic setting will help support the development of one's academic life, an early career faculty member should look for several features of the environment. The most basic elements include the presence of a mentor or mentors to help guide and some basic resources necessary to complete the academic work of the faculty member, e.g., access to a laboratory, access to a methodologist or quantitative expert, access to patient populations, access to students, and the like. Collaborative colleagues will enrich the academic environment further. If the productivity and workload expectations are rigorous but reasonable, and if there is a supervisor or even an opinion leader who values one's work, then the environment may well be sufficient. If there is a special aspect of an environment that is more important than all of the rest, in my view, it is whether there is a positive culture of curiosity, exploration, opportunity, and forgiveness that allows faculty members to learn, to expand their expertise, and to take on new responsibilities. One caveat: if the constellation of duties undertaken by the faculty member is not well-thought through, even the optimal academic environment will not support academic success. Carefully evaluating what is possible in the pairing of a faculty member and the institution/institutional role is therefore essential.

Beyond thinking about the context of one academic program or one organization, it is also valuable to entertain the possibility of making certain key moves over the course of one's professional life. These moves may occur within an institution, for instance, in seeking a new leadership role, or involve transitioning to a new faculty post at a new institution. Both kinds of change can be disruptive, and no one recommends "job-hopping." That said, intentional and well-judged moves both can bring immense opportunities for faculty members as well as the institutional environments in which they serve.

> *Far and away the best prize that life has to offer is the chance to work hard at work worth doing.*

> Theodore Roosevelt

The profession of academic medicine requires constant sustenance and renewal. For academic faculty, it is a time in history that holds the greatest promise in terms of scientific discovery, clinical innovation, educational advances, mutualism with other societal stakeholders, and true leadership. Each individual entering academic medicine can anticipate an exceptional career—one that is rich and exciting professionally and fulfilling personally. Our profession is nevertheless fragile. Resource concerns, erosion of the public trust, and inadequate numbers of people entering and remaining in scientific and clinical careers, in particular, threaten academic medicine. The significance of the fragility does not pertain to the interests of individual institutions or what may be perceived as petty concerns of "guild" subspecialties or disciplines—the real meaning is far greater because the consequences reach forward to the future. Our capacity to better the lives of people throughout the world, and shape the health of their children, will be lessened if academic medicine is allowed to languish. More positively stated, though it has been in existence for less than a century, the modern model of academic medicine has already brought about enduring good for humankind and, though the specific configuration of organizations may evolve, its value is certain to continue.

Inspiring exceptional young physicians and scientists, supporting them as they find their professional "calling," and fostering their development in academic medicine, taken together, therefore represent sincere commitments for our field. I said at the beginning of this chapter that academic medicine exists to help humanity, but it exists too because of the people who have committed their lives to it. For this reason, I end this initial chapter of *The Academic Medicine Handbook: A Guide to Achievement and Fulfillment for Academic Faculty* with a statement of appreciation for our early career colleagues, individuals who have already sacrificed and accomplished much and are choosing to join the authors of this volume on a professional path in academic medicine. We welcome

Words to the Wise
- Consider the five missions of academic medicine—where do your interests, strengths, and commitments fit?
- Take a good look at your colleagues and mentors: What can you learn from their career choices? What can you learn from their successes and failures?
- What practical skills do you need to progress in your career?
- How does your department compare with other departments nationally?
- What future do you envision in academic medicine?

Ask Your Mentor or Colleagues
- What kind of academic setting might be best for me?
- How can I prepare myself for the everyday duties of a new career in academic medicine?
- What are my strengths? Do I have limitations that I should try to remedy or compensate for?
- What are the predictable choice-points in an academic career path?
- Who else should I be talking with to help me think about my career and professional growth?

you to this endeavor, the work of imagining and creating a better future—and we thank you for stepping forward.

Reference

1. Roberts LW, Hilty DM. Approaching your academic career. In: Roberts LW, Hilty DM, editors. Handbook of career development in academic psychiatry and behavioral sciences. Arlington, VA: American Psychiatric Press, Inc; 2006. p. 3–10.

How to Build the Foundation for a Successful Career in Academia

Upinder Singh and Linda M. Boxer

It is the ultimate goal for many who go to medical or graduate school—joining the faculty ranks of an academic institution. For many, this seems an uphill battle, and financial, social, and life-style pressures are causing increasing number of graduates to abandon this goal. However, such a goal remains attainable, worth-while, and desirable and offers a challenging career filled with great rewards. A career in academic medicine is never routine or boring and provides enormous flexibility, yet enough intellectual stimulation and opportunities for growth to sustain interest and excitement for a lifetime.

In this chapter we outline some strategies that can pave the path to success while keeping in mind that each academic physician will have a unique and personal journey. Some factors that predict success are so obvious as to seem formulaic and repetitive, but still deserve discussion. Absolute requirements for the job are (1) possessing motivation and willingness to work hard, (2) being focused on goals in an efficient and organized manner that allows one to set priorities and achieve measurable success in them, (3) being prepared to network in one's field and obtain funding, and (4) having

L.M. Boxer, M.D., Ph.D. (✉)
Department of Medicine, Stanford University,
269 Campus Drive, Stanford, CA, USA
e-mail: lboxer@stanford.edu

© Springer International Publishing Switzerland 2016
L.W. Roberts (ed.), *The Associate Professor Guidebook*,
DOI 10.1007/978-3-319-28001-1_2

adequate protected time and aligning with the goals of the department and institution. Other skills are more nuanced and not so immediately obvious and relate to the ability to get the first academic job and to grow and mature in the position. These skills include the ability to deal with challenges and take risks and to understand one's strengths and weaknesses and learn from mistakes. Additionally, the ability to find mentors for different aspects of one's career and to be flexible enough to accommodate new opportunities and challenges is key to continued professional development and satisfaction.

Is This the Right Faculty Position?

In searching for a faculty position, a key predictor of future success is alignment of one's goals with those of the department and institution. Determine what an institution values and whether those priorities fit your short- and long-term goals. If your interests are not in line with the institutional vision, do not take a position just because you are enamored by the aura of the institution. Before accepting a faculty position, it is critical to agree with your chief or chair on how your effort will be divided among the three major academic missions of research, clinical care, and teaching. You will most likely spend significantly more time in one of the three missions. Likewise, the faculty position will be structured with a major focus on one of the missions. To accept a position that is not designed to allow you to spend the preponderance of your time on the mission that is of most importance to you and your career development is a recipe for disappointment and failure. In your discussions on the faculty position, be clear about the expectations that the chief or the chair has for what constitutes success. Spend the time to develop a realistic budget for your research needs for at least the first 3 years, and negotiate with the chief or the chair for this support. You will also need salary support during this time. Ask to see the offer in writing and make certain it is clear. Do not be afraid to ask for the resources and protected time that you need.

Once at the right place, finding colleagues who have similar aspirations will provide the essential intellectual support needed to develop your own scholarship. We do not live in a vacuum and certainly cannot succeed in one. Getting adequate support to develop your scholarship (protected time and resources being two important considerations) are key factors, as are clear expectations of how your time as a new faculty member will be spent (e.g., what proportion will be research, clinical, teaching, administrative). Many early-career faculty fall into the trap of overcommitting to too many service tasks early in their careers. The desire to be a good citizen is laudable, but the necessity to protect one's time during the early years of establishing a research program cannot be overstated.

Establishing Your Identity

Your research mentor has been a great guide for you and helped you develop as a scientist, writer, thinker, manager, and maybe even leader. However, as in all relationships, there is a time when some important and tough conversations must occur.

> Your angle: I am going out into the world and need to establish my scientific identity and I want to talk about how I will separate from you—what scientific projects would be yours and what work will be mine?
> Your mentor's angle: Great! I am excited for you to begin your own career. But your work has been some of the best in my lab—I am not sure how much of it I can give to you!

In the ideal world, the mentor's and trainee's goals, visions, and plans are completely aligned, but in the real world, where science is tough, funding difficult, and the competitive spirit drives all of us, the issue of separation and differentiation can often be challenging. To avoid misunderstandings, the best approach is to (1) have frank and honest conversations, (2) broach the topic early, (3) set up expectations on both sides, and (4) have regular follow-up. Another consideration is to have a specific time period when you are still working closely with a mentor but you are pursuing an independent project. This can be best accomplished when you have independent funding and will depend on the collaborative and collegial nature of your mentor. Keep in mind that science is difficult to predict. Even if your mentor and you agree to divide work, eventually your mentor's projects may collide with yours. Be prepared for this situation, but do not let fear of it hold you back from tackling the best and most interesting scientific questions. If your mentor has taught you well, you are prepared with the skills to be a friendly colleague, collaborator, and even competitor!

One special consideration is when you take a faculty position at the same institution as your mentor. Although such an arrangement has many advantages (e.g., you are already familiar with the environment, have scientific colleagues around you whom you know, can easily set up your own lab, and it is easier on you and your family not to move across the country), one disadvantage is continued association with your former mentor. In the eyes of your colleagues, will you be a new faculty colleague or simply the great senior postdoc of your mentor? This perception is not absolute and can be overcome, but you will have to make and follow a plan to overcome this perception successfully. Keep in mind that this separation is not just for the sake of your ego—it is for the sake of your career. When the time arrives for decisions on promotion and tenure, you will be judged on how you differentiated from your former mentor and whether you have established a research program that is unique, independent, and additive to the program of your mentor. In other words, what do you bring to the table that your mentor did not?

Setting Priorities and Focusing on Them

Once you have navigated the first few busy (and stressful!) years of life as a new faculty member, your thoughts will soon turn to the next steps—reappointment, promotion, and tenure. Have a discussion with your chief or chair on the criteria for reappointment and promotion. Different faculty lines are designed to emphasize each of the three academic missions, and the requirements for promotion will differ among the lines. You have previously made certain to enter the line that is the best fit for your goals and interests. Therefore, the criteria for promotion will likely align with your priorities. Once you have an understanding of the criteria for promotion, ask your mentors for their advice and feedback on what your priorities should be. Know the metrics on which you will be judged so that you can determine your readiness for and success in being promoted. Get as many perspectives as possible—ask, ask, ask. Ask those around you who have recently navigated this hurdle, ask mentors and supervisors what areas you should prioritize, and ask scientific colleagues for their insight and guidance. Among the abundance of advice you receive, common themes will emerge—keep those in mind as you set your goals and priorities.

It is very important to have protected time during your first several years on the faculty. Protected time will allow you to develop your scholarship, clinical practice, and/or teaching. When you are asked to take on a new project or assignment, consider how this work will help you attain your goals. Although some good citizenship activities are desirable and necessary, it is not reasonable to expect an early-career faculty member to engage heavily in these types of activities. With the advice and support of your mentors, determine which activities will be most beneficial for your career development without taking too much time away from your academic mission endeavors. Be focused and merciless about committing to new assignments or projects. Will they help or hinder you in your long-term goals? Taking on new projects that will ultimately help you is not being selfish—it is being smart.

Mentors, Mentors, and More Mentors

The importance of mentors as key predictors of success cannot be overstated. Academic medicine is complex, and listening to the advice of others who know how to negotiate the course will help ensure your success. You cannot have too many mentors, but do not expect them to seek you out. Go and find them. Keep in mind that you will need mentors for many aspects of your academic life—three areas that are the most obvious are research, clinical, and teaching. However, academic physicians also need and benefit from mentors in other areas—maintaining work–life balance, writing well and effectively, public speaking, and so on. It is valuable to have a mentoring team—one mentor does not have to fill all these varied roles. Keep in mind that your need for mentoring will also change over time, and the input and guidance you needed as a new faculty member will be vastly different from the guidance you need as you take on leadership roles. A good place to start in the search for mentors is with your chief or chair and/or your assigned mentor. Several of your mentors will likely be at your institution, but do not limit your mentorship support to colleagues at the same institution. For example, you may need to identify a mentor for your research from investigators in the same research area as yours, and it is quite possible that there will be no one at your home institution in your research field. Your research mentor from your time as a trainee may be able to assist with finding a mentor at another institution. Many institutions offer formal training in teaching skills, which is a valuable resource. It may be possible to identify a mentor to assist with developing your teaching abilities from among the faculty who participate in the training program. As you engage in clinical care, you will likely identify more senior clinical faculty who can serve as mentors and role models.

The best mentors provide honest feedback and advice, pointing to areas for improvement as well as helping you navigate the maze of academic medicine. A mentor who can identify areas for improvement and provide support and advice during the process is very skilled, and you will be fortunate to have such mentors. Stay flexible and be open-minded—many informal mentoring relationships can develop with senior colleagues. Although one does not often consider the need for support and advice on how to become a mentor as one begins a career in academic medicine, mentorship is an important requirement that will develop as you start to work with trainees in research and/or clinical care. One often unrecognized but great benefit to having wonderful mentors is that they can help you develop your mentoring skills. What aspects of a mentor were fantastic; what other habits were less than ideal? Look back at your experience and learn from it. Take the best of what you experienced and contribute to the next generation by being a great mentor. Many faculty members find the process of mentoring and developing early-career colleagues to be one of the most rewarding aspects of a career in academic medicine.

"Tooting Your Own Horn": Be Your Own Best Advocate

As scientists we are often taught to be modest—for example, analyze the data carefully, do not overcall your results, and do not be too broad and generalize beyond what this experiment shows. Although that approach works well in science, it can also hinder you when it is time for you to "sell" yourself. Remember that although your mentor, chief or chair, and other colleagues may do their best to promote you, the person who can best "pitch your product" is you. You need to be your own best advocate. Your job is to do great science, be a good mentor, communicate your data effectively and energetically, and network well with colleagues and collaborators. In addition, you need to keep track of what you have done for the institution (e.g., invited seminars, teaching responsibilities, committees, clinical work, mentoring students) and have that data for your supervisor. Having a systematic way to keep track of what you have contributed to the academic mission of your institution is key. You must toot your own horn—or at least provide the data to your chair so that he or she can toot a horn on your behalf!

I Do Not Look Like Other Faculty Members

The special challenges of being a faculty member as an underrepresented minority or a woman deserve mention. Identifying people whom we look like or to whom we aspire to emulate are important factors in shaping our thoughts about our potential. Seeing women faculty who have successful academic careers, handle work–life balance, and succeed in leadership positions gives the younger generation of women confidence that they too can have this career and be successful at it. For an underrepresented minority faculty member, the importance of finding others who look like him or her or have similar cultural backgrounds is also essential. As with many situations, success breeds success. An institution that has shown the commitment to recruit and retain underrepresented minority and women faculty members will have greater success with recruiting new faculty members in these categories. The awareness of the importance of having a rich, blended faculty at all ranks has been steadily increasing, and most nationally ranked institutions have special programs focused on the recruitment and retention of faculty who are women and underrepresented minorities.

What About My Significant Other?

It is now the norm that recruitment of a faculty member will involve assistance with career opportunities for his or her significant other. It may be a dual recruitment into the same department or different departments at the academic institution or help with locating an appropriate position in the area. This recruitment issue is particularly challenging not only for the couple but also for the institution. Many academic institutions have a person or an office to assist with issues related to dual-career couples. A significant question for the faculty applicant is when to raise this topic. As a candidate for a position, you should not be asked whether you have a significant other or family. You need to determine the appropriate time to begin this discussion. It may be reasonable to discuss this topic with the chair or the chief at the second visit or at the time you receive a formal offer. You and your significant other should decide in advance what assistance is needed, what kinds of positions would be appropriate for the other member of the couple, and what compromises you are each willing to accept. Dual-career couples face challenges at every stage of their training and career as they move forward in their professional lives. They may undergo a number of moves to different institutions, and these moves are often driven by the career of one member of the couple. How to balance the effect of a move on the career of the other member of the couple is difficult and must be handled with sensitivity on the part of all involved. This is another area in which mentors can be very helpful, especially those mentors who are members of dual-career couples themselves.

When Mistakes Happen

As accomplished as you are for winning the search for the faculty position, you will have areas of weakness or limitations that can be worked on and improved, just as everyone has. It is helpful to ask your mentors and others who know you well in different settings to assist you in evaluating your strengths and areas that require improvement. As you begin to work on your weaknesses, do not neglect your strengths. These are the personal characteristics that got you to where you are now and serve as the foundation of your success—do not neglect them, but enhance them and add to them. These can continue to be built upon, and you want to maintain them as areas that are strong for you. Once you have identified some limitations or weaknesses, work with your mentors on strategies to deal with them or to turn them into strengths. As an example, stubbornness is usually identified as a trait that is limiting, but you can learn to develop this trait into persistence, which is much more useful and can be a positive force.

As an early-career faculty member, you will feel the need to appear confident and knowledgeable. We all hope that each step along the path of an academic career will be filled with successes, but you will undoubtedly make mistakes along the way. You may identify a mistake or someone else may point it out to you. In either case, the best approach is to admit the mistake and work with your mentors to determine what you can learn from it. With this knowledge you can move forward and avoid making a similar mistake. The most worrisome aspect of mistakes is to fail to learn from them and to continue to err in the same way. Understanding your strengths and weaknesses and learning from your mistakes are crucial to continued personal and professional growth. To paraphrase a famous quote: those who cannot learn from failure are condemned to repeat it.

Continue to Take Risks

What brought you to where you are now was the ability to take scientific risks, think in new ways, and ask the big and important scientific questions. Creativity is valued in academic medicine, and success often results from the use of novel approaches. Once you are in a faculty role, it is important not to lose this perspective. Although the initial focus may be in pursuing some safer route, one needs to be creative, willing to try new approaches, and open to new experiences. Having a mixture of high-risk/high-reward projects in addition to those that are likely to succeed is generally the best approach. The safer projects are those that are guaranteed to get papers published and lay the foundation for grants and funding. Advice from an experienced research mentor will be valuable in assessing the balance of research projects in your portfolio. The colleagues that surround us are often catalysts for initiating new projects, and although having plans for your research program is important, it is also important to be ready to take on new opportunities when they present themselves. As we take on each new challenge, we learn from it, grow, improve, and develop.

With your mentors, you will chart a path for success as a new faculty member. Throughout your career, however, you will be presented with opportunities that you did not foresee or necessarily seek. Although these may not be part of your plans for career development, it is essential to remain open to new possibilities. You can assess a new opportunity with the assistance of your mentors and determine whether it is one you choose to pursue. It is important to appraise whether you will thrive in the new role or option, and how it will affect the other areas of your work, including research, clinical care, and teaching. It is beneficial to take on challenges and to learn from them. Clearly, the most important goal of an early-career faculty member is to focus on the three major missions and make the strongest case possible for promotion. Therefore, any new opportunity must be judged in this context.

Work–Life Balance: Do Not Ignore It!

The importance of work–life balance and making time to "recharge" cannot be overstated. Remember, this is a marathon, not a sprint. Everyone needs to have time to recharge, both intellectually and emotionally. People are most creative when they have the mental freedom to think, explore, and ponder. Stifling the creative spirit by not allowing oneself to recharge is a common mistake among young scientists. There cannot be perfect work–life balance in every day, every week, or even every month—months with a grant deadline, for example. A careful self-assessment should be performed on a routine basis so that the balance of work and life is maintained. See what others are doing to maintain some level of harmony and find examples you want—or do not want—to emulate. Then figure out your personal solution. A career in academic medicine, particularly as a new faculty member, comes with substantial pressures and stress. You will need to develop methods to handle stress and maintain a healthy lifestyle. Not all approaches to stress management are healthy. You can learn from your mentors and colleagues how they minimize stress and maintain a healthy balance between work and other aspects of their life. A career in academic medicine can be very rewarding. You have intellectual freedom and can make a positive impact in a number of areas. As a new faculty member, your entire career lies ahead of you. With hard work and support and advice from senior colleagues, you are off to a great start.

Conclusion

It takes an enormous amount of motivation, hard work, perseverance, and determination to reach the point where one is offered a faculty position. However, the hard work is not done, and the next steps (e.g., getting your scholarly program established and productive) are often just as challenging. Apply the same strategies and approaches that got you this far: be efficient; commit to the time it will take to build your career; make plans, including a timeline for obtaining research grants and writing papers; and network with others in your field by going to meetings and interacting with the leaders in your area of scholarship. Your mentors will provide support and advice, but you must be committed to building your career and spending the time that is required for this. When you are at work, maintain your focus on the tasks at hand. Learn to be as efficient as possible, seeking guidance and training with efficiency if necessary. Determine what is important for your career success. Make a timeline for the submission of grants supported by strong preliminary data and for the preparation of manuscripts. Be certain to attend important meetings in your field of scholarship, and make an effort to meet the leaders in the field. Your research mentor can help facilitate these meetings and your invitations to meetings to present your research. Promotion requires visibility in your area of scholarship, and investigators in the field will be asked to critique your scholarship and assess your likelihood for continued success. Maintain time for yourself and your family—and keep your creative spirits flowing. Most important, take time to reflect on why you love the job of academic medicine and enjoy the process!

Words to the Wise
- You cannot have too many mentors.
- Be certain to obtain sufficient protected time to develop scholarship.
- Set priorities and focus on them.
- Make certain your goals fit with those of the department and the institution.
- Success requires motivation and hard work.
- Understand your strengths and weakness and learn from your mistakes.
- Do not be afraid to take risks.
- Do not neglect other aspects of your life; work–life balance is the key to long-term success.

Ask Your Mentor or Colleagues
- Give me honest feedback—how do you think I am doing?
- What are the next steps for my career development?
- What was the biggest mistake you made in your first position?
- What was your best decision in your first position?
- What is the best advice you can give me at this point in my career?
- How do you maintain a balance between work and the rest of your life and how do you deal with stress?

How to Be Organized and Manage Time

3

Robert K. Jackler

> *Time keeps on slippin', slippin', slippin' Into the future.*
>
> Steve Miller Band

The great majority of medical school faculty members begin their faculty service with an abundance of motivation, drive, and ability. Among those who fail to fully achieve their career aspirations, the most common reason is an inability to effectively manage their time. Of all the skills needed to achieve success in academic medicine, perhaps most essential is the ability to achieve balance among innumerable commitments to enable at least passable success in all domains.

Avoiding the Overcommitment Trap

Success as an academic physician requires demarcating protected time for scholarship and defending it from intrusion by other duties. If an academic physician demonstrates ability in any arena (clinical, educational, administrative), he or she will inevitably be

R.K. Jackler, M.D. (✉)
Department of Otolaryngology—Head and Neck Surgery,
Stanford University Medical Center, 801 Welch Road,
Stanford, CA, USA
e-mail: jackler@stanford.edu

© Springer International Publishing Switzerland 2016
L.W. Roberts (ed.), *The Associate Professor Guidebook*,
DOI 10.1007/978-3-319-28001-1_3

invited to take on more and more such responsibilities. For example, if one has made worthwhile contributions to a task force or *ad hoc* committee, rest assured that academic physician will receive at least twice as many such invitations in the subsequent year. Both medical schools and their affiliated medical centers have an insatiable need for physician engagement in administrative activities.

The foremost cause of overcommitment in academic medicine is the tendency of early-career faculty to be "too nice" when it comes to seeing patients. In eagerness to build a clinical practice, the inclination is to accept every overbooked patient, consult request, and procedure invitation. The gradual squeezing out of academic time by burgeoning clinical activities is by far the leading cause of "infant mortality" among promising young physician-scientists. Aside from the natural tendency of many physicians to gravitate toward patient care, economic incentives often come into play. Many university compensation plans reward clinical revenue generation more generously than time spent in research or education. In many fields, a majority of new faculty members find that their clinical role expands to the degree that they become primarily clinicians and teachers with little time remaining for scholarly endeavors.

Simply put, the most important word in an academic physician's lexicon is *no*. Learning to graciously decline proffered opportunities in a manner that does not diminish the inviter's opinion of you is a crucial survival skill. One useful strategy is to thank the inviter for considering you, acknowledging that the task is most worthwhile, but that to accept the offer would mean giving up another worthy activity. It is essential to be polite, firm, and resolute in declining because those seeking your involvement will often attempt to negotiate lower levels of engagement which, once accepted, will inevitably follow a slippery slope to greater and greater levels of time commitment. It is far better to one's reputation as a faculty member to say no up front than it is to accept an assignment and be unable to fully meet its requirements.

The "Peter Principle" permeates the culture of academic medicine. If an academic physician is both very busy and very effective, he or she will inevitably be asked to engage in more and more responsibilities. The fortunate paradox is that if one is widely recognized to be very busy, it makes it that much easier for others to accept one's polite refusal of offers for more work. The take-home point is that it is wise and prudent to have others see you as heavily committed, but not so overcommitted that they would not consider offering you an opportunity that would further your career goals. A corollary to this principle is knowing when and how to disengage from a lower priority commitment to free up time to enable you to accept an activity of higher priority. Usually the best rule of thumb is transparency—an honest explanation of one's reasons for withdrawal will usually be well received.

Experienced academic physicians can offer helpful advice on managing commitments. This subject is one of the highest-priority subjects to seek mentorship (and protection) from your division chief and/or department chair. They can even provide political "cover": "My Chair asked that I not see clinic patients on my research days." "My Chief does not want me to take on any more committee assignments at this time."

Making Effective Use of the Interstices of the Day

Day: A period of twenty-four hours, mostly misspent.

Ambrose Bierce

Only a fraction of each working day is spent engaged in patient care, teaching, research, or administration. In aggregate, the interstices of the day add up to a considerable opportunity to enhance your productivity. Examples of these time fragments include the wait between patient visits and operating room cases, anticipating the start of a meeting or a class, and time spent on hold. It also includes transit time such as waiting for elevators and in cafeteria lines. In total, this often-underutilized time resource is likely to amount to some 15–20 % of the workday [1]. It is important to first acknowledge that these time intervals are often used for the worthy purposes of socialization with coworkers or catching a few moments of relaxation. However, if they are spent productively, they may ultimately facilitate more time with family or on recreational activities.

It helps to have readily available "bite-sized" pieces of work to fill in the day's gaps. In the modern era, managing the electronic mail inbox, a few messages at a time, lessens the need for a lengthy session to handle a sizeable accumulation. In the clinical arena, between time can be used to complete charting or dictation and manage an electronic medical record inbox. Interstices are also a good opportunity to absorb a few research papers, review/edit a manuscript, or return a phone call or two. Meal breaks, when not used for meetings or socialization, are an opportunity to accomplish some worthwhile tasks to lighten the load at the end of the day.

Walter Dandy, an eminent Johns Hopkins neurosurgeon of the first half of the twentieth century, used to take the train from Baltimore to Chicago and back merely to provide time to catch up on academic writing. Many of today's academic physicians spend a considerable amount of time either in airplanes or in terminals waiting for airplanes. This represents a precious opportunity to work on scholarly projects in a focused and uninterrupted manner. For example, the present chapter was written on an airplane while travelling to and from a family trip over the winter holidays. The reader, no doubt, joins my wife who made the observation that had I better managed my time, this work would not have been necessary.

Most physicians have daily commutes by car. Using hands-free devices, one may use this time as a prime opportunity to conduct telephone discussions. It is also an opportunity to make use of digital audio recordings that are available of continuing medical education programs, grand rounds, and scientific meeting proceedings.

Limiting Interruptions and Distractions

Happiness can only be found if you can free yourself of all other distractions.

Saul Bellow

Some people can only be productive in a linear environment—that is to say, working in a quiet place, on one thing at a time, with neither interruptions nor distractions. Clearly, such individuals are not well suited for a life in academic medicine. However, even those relatively tolerant of a nonlinear work environment find too many interruptions and distractions to be a source of stress that can lead to job dissatisfaction and even "burnout." It is essential to train staff members to batch lower priority items needing attention rather than continuously interrupting you. Pagers, cell phones, and texting are helpful tools in modern medicine, but if they are used in an undisciplined manner, they can tempt staff to offload problems onto faculty (at their convenience) rather than organize them to enhance faculty efficiency. Working with one's clinic staff and academic administrative assistant to establish guidelines for how and when to interrupt is time well spent. Use of electronic mail for lower priority issues enables the academic physician to address them at his or her convenience.

While academic physicians have little choice but to learn tolerance for the chaotic work of clinical medicine, their scholarly endeavors necessitate a quiet environment with minimal disturbances. This is the reason so many papers and grant proposals are written in the evening or over weekends at home, at times to the detriment of family life. Whenever practical, establish a well-defended portion of each week for scholarly activities that will not be disturbed save for truly urgent reasons.

Faculty members who make themselves readily available at all times will tend to see this privilege used more and more heavily. If one is easy to reach, colleagues and staff will tend to follow the path of least resistance and hand off issues needing attention. One secret of avoiding excessive entanglements is to selectively make it harder to be reached. One does not want to be perceived as the most convenient recipient of transferred workload. For example, tell the clinic staff to batch all nonurgent calls and messages until clinical days. When a breakthrough call is received that could have waited for a clinic day, push back gently, but firmly, lest the interruptions to academic time inevitably proliferate.

One useful device to limit distractions is the closed office door. If one's staffs understand that a closed door signals that one is busy and that interruptions should be limited to compelling cause, they will help to defend one's time for academic activities. Another useful demarcation is time clearly indicated as "in the lab." An understanding among clinical and academic staff that time dedicated to research is sacrosanct will tend to keep it so. It helps to set parameters among the staff, residents, and fellows about the circumstances under which such time limits can be breached. At times staff and trainees will inevitably intrude for manifestly unnecessary reasons. Effectively managing trivial intrusions of precious academic time is crucial. A polite, but firm, explanation about how difficult it is to finish an experiment, write a paper, or complete a grant with multiple interruptions that could have waited usually hits the mark.

Multitasking: Beneficial or Deleterious?

For better or worse, multitasking has become a fact of life in academic medicine. It used to be considered impolite for a medical student to read a newspaper during a lecture, even seated in the back row of the lecture hall with the paper folded discretely on his or her lap. Times have certainly changed. The proliferation of portable digital devices such as cell phones, notebook computers, and tablets have fundamentally altered the cultural acceptability of multitasking. Many residents and faculty attend grand rounds with computers open in front of them, which they engage with frequent bursts of rapid fire typing. It is a losing battle to attempt to regulate or forbid multitasking. It is helpful to encourage trainees to engage in content-relevant multitasking (e.g., PubMed rather than Facebook). Experience gleaned through directing random Socratic questions at learners makes it clear that at least some are fully capable of absorbing multiple simultaneous information streams while still effectively tracking the educational activity while others are clearly distracted and unengaged.

This phenomenon is not entirely generational; almost all leaders at a university's multiday dean's retreats use their laptops throughout. Multitasking at lectures, meetings, and retreats has become so endemic that it is now virtually the cultural norm. One consequence is that while lecture rooms used to fill from either the front or the back, today the most precious real estate in a lecture hall is the discrete back corner of the room with access to power plugs on the side wall.

To some degree, the ability to pay attention and comprehend multiple inputs simultaneously is variable among individuals. If you have this ability, then using it judiciously will be of benefit.

Academic life is full of opportunities to multitask. Multi-participant teleconferences are ideal because no one needs to know you are multitasking (unless you type too vigorously).

Planning and Organizing

I skate to where the puck is going to be, not where it has been.

Wayne Gretzky

A minute spent on planning is worth an hour later. It pays time dividends to organize one's efforts to build in quality up front rather than having to reconfigure one's efforts later. For example, when preparing a grant submission, scan the technical requirements and format instructions before starting. At best, mistakes can be a source of delay and wasted effort; at worst, a reason for disqualification. Similarly, when preparing a manuscript, consult the journal's instructions for authors. Reconfiguring a completed manuscript can lead to considerable time lost.

Although it is no one's favorite thing to do, spend time learning the basics of regulatory compliance in areas relevant to one's work. This includes human and animal experimental protocols, management of private health information (HIPAA), and the basics of budgeting and personnel management. Failure to organize research in a compliant manner can lead to serious consequences and may disqualify one's work from publication. Most universities provide expert guidance on such matters, and this is best sought in advance.

Most physicians hate to complete the all-too-common, mandatory training modules, especially when they have to be repeated on a yearly basis. (It is ironic that today's physicians have to be repeatedly retested on regulatory matters but not on medical knowledge crucial to patient care.) In a worthwhile time-saving maneuver, some online modules allow the academic physician to skip the didactics and go straight to taking the test. If one has completed the material before, chances are pretty good that he or she can make it over the passing bar. Some training modules require spending at least a minimal amount of time on the didactic portion. This is one reason why modern computers enable opening multiple windows.

Managing Deadlines

Some deadlines are genuine, while others are relative points in time. Examples of firm deadlines are grant submission dates and warnings about suspension of medical staff privileges due to incomplete medical records. The firmness of publishing deadlines are variable. The "deadline" for submitting a book chapter is notoriously soft. Multi-authored textbooks typically have only half to two thirds of chapters by the first deadline. Textbook chapters tend to be of lower priority, to be completed as time allows. It is human nature to believe that a less-pressured time will come soon, affording an opportunity to conveniently catch up. Of course, this is usually a false perception. Procrastination can lead to a feeling of continual crisis management punctuated by late nights and weekends.

Optimizing Scholarship

Choose academic projects carefully. Just because something is easy to study does not mean it is worthwhile to study. Much time is wasted on projects that lack originality or even scientific value. When considering a project, always ask the "so what" question: If I knew the results of the project today, how much better off would I be? If the proposal lacks impact, do not waste precious academic time on it. As most worthwhile research has a substantial probability of failure, so it is also important to recognize early when a research project is unfruitful, cut one's losses, and move on.

When conceptualizing a study, seek advice from colleagues on the soundness of the hypothesis and on the optimal study design. Obtain statistical consultation during the design phase, before obtaining data, especially for clinical trials. Most university medical centers have clinical trial specialists and data managers to assist clinical studies and hold training courses to teach these skills. The academic physician who has not been trained in clinical trial design and management may consider the time invested in becoming more knowledgeable well spent.

Most faculty members conduct research and author scholarly publications together with medical and graduate students, residents, fellows, and postdocs. From the perspective of a faculty member's career development, this is both an essential teaching role and an opportunity to amplify one's scholarship. Although trainees are essential to furthering one's research goals, writing a paper with trainees often takes more, rather than less, time to complete. Because trainees are inexperienced, it is best to give them an outline and carefully monitor their progress.

The ability to write well is key to success in an academic career. Authoring a scientific communication is one task best not done in haste. It is better to take one's time to craft a paper that is free from errors and possesses both clarity and persuasiveness in its arguments. It is wise to put down your completed draft and look at it again with fresh eyes after some time has gone by. Writing which seemed polished at the time you wrote it may show its flaws after time has dulled your familiarity with it. Before finalizing, ask a number of colleagues to review your paper and provide constructive criticism. Before submitting for publication, ask yourself the key question: "if I look back on this paper in twenty years, will I still be proud of it?"

In manuscript preparation, interminable revision loops can be a huge time sink. It is sometimes better to sit down together to write as a team. In multi-authored papers, great care must be taken to avoid version confusion and having to repeat already completed work. Naming the draft with a date or version number helps to keep track. Bibliographic management software is a worthwhile tool in managing references with multiple authors. Keep in mind that journals require each author to sign the copyright transmittal notice. Given the typical travel schedules of academic collaborators, it is best to not leave this task for last minute.

In building a CV in anticipation of eventual promotion, it is important to realize that not all scholarship is valued equally. Many university promotion committees place little value on writing textbook chapters or even entire textbooks, considering them evidence of teaching rather than scholarship. Early-career faculty members ought not become bogged down contributing numerous chapters at the expense of undertaking original research that makes a scientific contribution.

When one's name is listed on a paper, that person has agreed to accept authorship responsibility. It behooves each author to spend the time needed to carefully check the manuscript for quality, validity, and veracity. If the published paper contains errors or transgresses publication ethics (e.g., failure to cite, redundant publication, plagiarism), each author shares responsibility, even if a coauthor contributed this section.

Early-career faculty members are often handed papers to review by more senior faculty. Whenever possible, the academic physician should submit the review under his or her own signature. This lets the journal editor know of one's availability as a reviewer. It is a misconception that journal editorial boards are drawn exclusively from famous leaders in the field. If an academic physician responds to the editors' requests promptly and submits thoughtful reviews, he or she has found the pathway to editorial service. Journals track peer reviewer performance and highly value timeliness, because a quick decision is much appreciated by manuscript authors.

Academic physicians are often invited to organize the scholarship of other academicians, such as in textbooks or special issues of journals. Because scholars are perpetually late, a prudent editor builds in a series of deadlines before the genuine one and sends out frequent reminders of progressively more strident tone. It is also wise to have a backup plan in place, typically an author willing to perform on short notice, for those who never submit.

Managing Clinical Responsibilities

Time is money.

Benjamin Franklin

The practice of medicine is the largest time commitment for most medical school faculty. The two most important principles in keeping clinical responsibilities from overwhelming all others are setting time boundaries and managing one's schedule so that one stays within scheduled time as much as possible. Academic practices have the disadvantage of having a fraction of patients who travel from a distance, making it impractical to break up visits into multiple sessions, as is often done in private practice. In large university clinics, scheduling is often done by staff members who are subject to persistent patient pressure to get an appointment but are remote from patients' discontent when they suffer long waits or hurried visits. Because unrealistic scheduling (e.g., a new patient with a complex history put in a 15-min slot) and systematic overbooking are endemic in academic medicine, time spent setting up a realistic outpatient clinic template is well worthwhile. A common example is that of a physician who is fully booked for a month with no slots preserved for urgent referrals, unanticipated revisits for acute illness, and pre- or post-procedure appointments, which is a recipe for dysfunctional levels of overbooking. It is prudent for the academic physician to work closely with practice management on a realistic schedule template and on motivating the managerial discipline to hold open an adequate number of slots to accommodate patients needing timely attention. Routinely reviewing one's schedule a week or 2 beforehand helps to identify unrealistic scheduling while there is still time to remediate the situation.

An obvious first principle of time management in outpatient clinics is starting on time. Learning how to manage challenging patients is at the core of academic practice. It has been said that two types of patients dominate university practices: "normal" people afflicted by complex disease and "difficult" people with relatively minor maladies. As the "highest level of appeal" for patients who have yet to find answers, it is the academic physician's job to provide them. Experienced physicians learn how to manage patients' questions in ways that are both satisfying and time efficient. For example, when a patient asks why a particular test has not been ordered or a type of treatment tried, it is common to engage in a lengthy discussion on the subject of indications and contraindications which can be received as "medical authority" and satisfy the patient. The elegantly simple reply "I did not recommend it because I did not think it would help you" sends a positive message of caring and, in many instances, succeeds in reassuring the patient. Because many such techniques are specialty specific, seek advice from experienced clinicians.

Much efficiency can be gained while maintaining the medical record. Writing a concise plan of what is expected for the next visit allows a quick review of the previous note to orient the physician upon active problems. In electronic systems, the earlier note can be propagated and modified for use during a new visit.

Personalized automated phrases and patient informational handouts are great time savers. In procedure notes, later review is expedited by including a "findings" section to extract key points. The anticipated next steps in the patient's management quickly emerge in the review of the earlier entry. While it is somewhat a matter of individual preference, bundling of dictation is not ideal. Memory of the encounter is freshest at the time of the visit, and incomplete charts tend to be put aside until well after memory of the visit has become somewhat hazy. Communicating with patients via e-mail is a double-edged sword. On one hand, it saves time by allowing routine medical questions to be answered conveniently and is notably more efficient than using the telephone. On the other hand, it gives the patient direct access to the physician for unsuitably complex and/or urgent questions or even administrative matters (e.g., "Please make me an appointment") more appropriately handled by office staff. It is helpful having a standard text block available to politely inform patients of your use guidelines for electronic mail.

Delegation: Effective Use of Staff

To be successful, a new academic physician has to learn quickly to work effectively with a team. Take the time to get to know every staff member personally and work to enfranchise staff in a shared mission of excellence—whether it is to deliver great patient care or to seek a cure for cancer. Always treat staff in a courteous and respectful manner and frequently show appreciation for jobs well done. If you are harsh or abrupt, it will create an unpleasant work culture, and staff will not give you their best effort. Working with an efficient staff is essential for a physician to be efficient.

Meet with your clinical and research teams regularly to set out goals and expectations. For major tasks, set timeline expectations and monitor progress regularly. Staff members learning their roles, and even those who are well trained, sometimes engage in "problem dumping." This is defined as passing the buck up the chain to the physician when the issue could actually have been resolved at a staff level. When this has become troublesome, as it inevitably will be from time to time, work with your managers to help counsel staff to better meet your expectations. It is worthwhile to spend time in preparing formal written reviews of staff performance and being frank about reasons for praise and opportunities for improvement.

It is important that staff members know how to reach you at all times and even more important that they learn to use this privilege appropriately. To minimize interruptions, provide clear guidelines for what is urgent and what can wait. In configuring the guidelines, it is better to tolerate some leakage of nonurgent matters than to have a truly urgent communication not reach you in a timely manner. Direct access to you is especially important when the person making the triage decision is not clinically trained. Be sure to set aside adequate time to expeditiously handle nonurgent matters that your staff has batched for you.

In the laboratory, work closely with those who support grant preparation and post-award management. Your valuable time should not be spent on routine accounting of lab expenses or on the process of purchasing equipment or supplies. The staff should be expected to support your material ordering and provide timely and informative tracking of expenses and resources remaining in your research fund.

Selectivity in Choosing Administrative Roles

All academic physicians are called upon to participate in administrative roles. Faculty members are often put in positions of authority in which they are responsible for managing people, tasks, and money despite the fact that they lack the training and experience that would be prerequisites in the business world. Taking a formal course in leadership training, as is available in many medical schools, is time well spent by early-career faculty.

Administrative service is time intensive. The first principle of keeping your time commitment in line is to keep small problems from becoming big ones by early and effective attention. A second is to find ways to prevent the myriad regulations inherent in modern medical centers and biomedical research from inhibiting quality patient care and innovative research, which often necessitates negotiating a compromise with compliance professionals rather than accepting their invariably conservative recommendations as edicts.

The pathway to administrative service usually commences with committee service for the school of medicine or medical center. Early-career faculty striving to establish themselves are well advised to avoid especially-time-consuming committee assignments, such as medical school admissions (due to time-intensive interviews and panel meetings) and the committees on human and animal research (numerous protocols to review and debate). Although committees are somewhat institutionally dependent, some good ones to begin with are quality of care, ambulatory care, curriculum reform, and time-limited ad hoc task forces focused on an issue relevant to one's research or clinical work.

Work–Life Balance

Working more does not always equal greater productivity; indeed, it can have the opposite effect. Unbalanced lifestyles can lead to dissatisfaction and, ultimately, burnout. Overwhelmed physicians become mechanical in their clinical role and are at risk for losing their passion for healing others. A stressed, irascible, and exhausted faculty member makes a poor role model for physicians in training. In scholarship, being overwhelmed stifles creativity and inventiveness. Avoiding burnout requires setting manageable limits and boundaries between work and domestic life. If you feel you are beginning to fall victim to burnout, seek counsel from your division chief, department chair, or other respected colleague to help provide perspective on ways of reestablishing your work–life balance. Formal psychological counseling on stress management may be worthwhile.

When an academic physician feels stagnant, pursuing a new line of research or adopting an emerging clinical technique may be reinvigorating. Taking a sabbatical leave with institutional support is a healthy way of retooling scholarly focus and reasserting control of one's schedule.

Words to the Wise
- Inability to manage time effectively is the most common reason academic physicians fail to achieve their career goals.
- It is essential to set and maintain boundaries to protect time for scholarly work.
- Successful academic faculty members avoid overcommitment by learning how to graciously say "no."
- The ability to delegate tasks to academic and clinical staff helps to offload workload.
- It is human nature to believe that a less pressured time will come soon, affording an opportunity to conveniently catch up. This is usually a false perception.
- In administrative tasks, the first principle is to keep small problems from becoming big ones by early and effective attention.

Ask Your Mentor or Colleagues
- How have you been able to say no to additional activities and responsibilities?
- What are your strategies for managing time?
- How do you balance professional demands against your personal life?

Reference

1. Tipping MD, Forth VE, O'Leary KJ, et al. Where did the day go? A time motion study of hospitalists. J Hosp Med. 2010;5:323–8.

Further Reading

Lowenstein SR. Tuesdays to write. A guide to time management in academic emergency medicine. Acad Emerg Med. 2009:165–7.

Fox WL. Dandy of Johns Hopkins. Baltimore: Williams & Wilkins; 1984.

Brunicardi FC, Hobson FL. Time management: a review for physicians. J Nat Med Assn. 1996;88:581–7.

Shanafelt TD, West CP, et al. Career fit and burnout among academic faculty. Arch Int Med. 2009;169:990–5.

Solomon J. How strategies for managing patient visit time affect physician job satisfaction: a quantitative analysis. J Gen Int Med. 2008;23:775–80.

Dyrbye LN, West CP, et al. Work/home conflict and burnout among academic internal medicine physicians. Arch Int Med. 2011;171 (online publication).

Papadakos PK. Electronic distraction: an unmeasured variable ipn modern medicine. Anesthesia News. 2011;37:11.

Pisano ED. Time management 101. Acad Radiol. 2001;8:768–70.

Thornburg LL, Glantz JC, Caprio TV, et al. Professional bankruptcy for the academic physician. J Grad Med Educ. 2010;2:485–7.

Gruber PJ. Idealism versus reality: the modern surgeon-scientist. Ann Thorac Surg. 2008;85:1151–2.

Chiu RCJ. The challenge of "Tending the Bridge". Ann Thorac Surg. 2008;85:1149–50.

Dugdale DC, Epstein R, Pantilat SZ. Time and the patient-physician relationship. J Gen Intern Med. 1999;14 Suppl 1:S34–40.

Mauksch LB, Dugdale DC, Dodson S, et al. Relationship, communication, and efficiency in the medical encounter: creating a clinical model from a literature review. Arch Intern Med. 2008;168: 1387–95.

Nuel JL. Interested in a career as a clinician scientist? Dis Models Mech. 2010;3:125–30.

How to Have a Healthy Life Balance as an Academic Physician

4

Christine Moutier

The well-being of physicians has personal, professional, and public health ramifications. A physician's personal health and well-being are not only vital to the individual physician and his or her family members and community but may also affect that physician's life professionally. Moreover, on a larger societal scale, physician wellness also likely serves a critical role in the delivery of high-quality healthcare. When physicians are unwell, the performance of healthcare systems can be negatively affected [1]. Good health and mental well-being contribute to the solid foundation on which physicians can be resilient in the face of challenge and optimally address the many stresses of professional life and clinical work. But even for those physicians who understand this connection and are motivated to improve their situation, the real rub comes in practical obstacles of time and energy. Limitations of time and energy are very real, and after the essential tasks of one's work and personal responsibilities are fulfilled, physicians may feel there is little time left to create change that could lead to improvement in health or well-being. This chapter will provide strategies to address this particularly vexing problem many academic physicians face: how to optimally balance work and personal life to enhance the outcome on both sides.

C. Moutier, M.D. (✉)

Department of Psychiatry, University of California, San Diego, School of Medicine, 9500 Gilman Drive, La Jolla, CA, USA

e-mail: cmoutier@ucsd.edu

© Springer International Publishing Switzerland 2016
L.W. Roberts (ed.), *The Associate Professor Guidebook*,
DOI 10.1007/978-3-319-28001-1_4

Physician Distress

The literature on physician and trainee distress has shown an association between various forms of distress and both professional commitment and clinical performance. The predicted shortfall of physicians in the workforce is compounded by continued concerns about job satisfaction and intention to leave the profession [2]. Burnout, depressive symptoms, and low quality of life are all too common among resident physicians and have been associated with negative effects on patient care including major medical and medication errors, suboptimal care practices, and decreased patient satisfaction with medical care [3]. Among medical students, burnout has been associated with lower levels of empathy and increased incidence of unprofessional behaviors such as cheating [4]. When burnout is severe and chronic (>12 months) even more severe forms of distress, such as suicidal ideation, occur at higher rates [5]. Unfortunately, physicians have higher rates of completed suicide than their age-matched nonphysician peers [6]. While suicide comprises a narrow and very extreme sequelae of underrecognized, untreated, or undertreated psychiatric illness, it is an important and tragic outcome along the continuum of physician distress.

Efforts in Medical Education

Undergraduate medical education promotes the concept of self-care as a physician's professional responsibility, teaches wellness strategies, attempts to destigmatize mental healthcare, and encourages help-seeking at appropriate times. In 2002 the accrediting body for U.S. medical schools, the Liaison Committee on Medical Education, mandated that medical schools prioritize student wellness by providing education related to well-being and stress management and regular opportunities to participate in activities that promote resilience and optimal physical and mental health. Graduate medical education similarly has made significant changes in the area of resident well-being, originally driven by the need to protect patient safety, but more recently with an integrated concern for both resident well-being and its interconnection with patient care. These efforts have specifically addressed resident sleep and fatigue with changes in the Accreditation Council for Graduate Medical Education regulations in 2003 and 2011 not only limiting work hours but also requiring the monitoring of resident well-being. Medical education and training may be a time when young physicians learn early habits (for good or for bad) and may be particularly sensitive to the informal curriculum of the profession, which has not always promoted the prioritizing of one's own well-being.

Conceptual Framework for Wellness

For a given individual, how does an everyday mishap (e.g., spilt milk) lead to a calm, even compassionate response on one day but provoke an irritable outburst on another? Imagine that the myriad of internal human factors (physiologic, psychological, spiritual) that culminate in the most mature intellectual, emotional, and behavioral response in the face of stress can be condensed into one substance, a fuel source if you will, which, if used fully by the mind and heart, lead to the most healthy, optimal, and likely ethical responses to the plethora of stressors that come up in every day personal and professional life of physicians. In a dynamic way, the day-to-day and even moment-to-moment thoughts, ideas, and responses to stress may be viewed in a model akin to a complex mechanical system. This system relies on an adequate fuel source to perform its functions in a streamlined way. In a similar way, an individual's responses are affected by the amount and quality of "reserve fuel" from which to draw. The human coping reservoir depends on positive input (inflow of fuel), negative input (outflow or loss of fuel), and the structure and characteristics of the reservoir itself [7] (see Fig. 4.1).

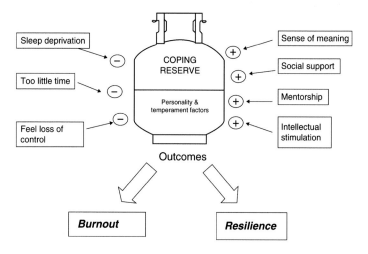

Fig. 4.1 Conceptual model of a coping reservoir. Adapted from [7]

Key Concepts
- *Flourishing*: Optimal state of human existence and functioning, cultivated over a period of time, that encompasses a sense of goodness, generativity, growth, and resilience. An area of study in the field of positive psychology.
- *Burnout*: A response to chronic occupational stress. Tends to occur when workload is high and sense of autonomy, control, and meaning in one's work is low. Consists of a triad of experiences: (1) emotional depletion, (2) sense of detachment, and (3) low sense of achievement.

Internal Structure and Characteristics of the Coping Reservoir

Academic physicians come to the profession of medicine with unique personal characteristics and therefore different strengths and weaknesses. Some are more intrinsically resilient than others and some are more prone to anxiety and depression. This intrinsic "sturdiness" versus "leakiness" of the reservoir is based on a variety of factors including genetics, early childhood, and current environmental factors, and temperament, such as optimism and neuroticism. Physicians tend to be highly driven, conscientious to obsessive, and relatively stoic. While these traits can be positive qualities in a physician, they can also lead to personal suffering.

Depleting Factors (Negative Inputs)

The following areas are common sources of depletion of the coping reservoir, but naturally there are as many unique drains on well-being and resilience as there are individuals.

1. *Stress*: The topic of stress encompasses a vast area and is an unavoidable reality of life for all. Early in medical training, curricular and academic rigors of medical school and residency are easily identified stressors; however, neither education nor stress ends with formal training. Physicians in practice must keep abreast of an ever-enlarging body of skills and knowledge while performing all of the tasks and responsibilities of a busy clinical practice. The struggle for some physicians to keep up-to-date may be squashed by the overwhelming demands of practice. This may be especially true for high-volume, solo, clinical practice environments. This struggle can lead to fears about one's competence on the one hand, or rationalization or even denial of one's deficiencies on the other. There are also common personal psychosocial events which physicians may experience at any age or stage of career. These include personal or family illness, divorce or the break-up of a relationship, death of a loved one, and/or financial problems. The convergence of personal crisis with the steady level of professional stress may lead to a decrement in overall well-being, and in this relatively decompensated state, coping strategies may then deteriorate into less adaptive ones. Maladaptive attempts to cope like using alcohol or drugs (prescription or illicit) obviously pose further risk, such as loss of judgment and legal and/or clinical ramifications. Another pathway that can challenge homeostatic well-being is the occurrence of professional crisis such as a particularly

difficult malpractice suit, interpersonal problems in the workplace, or the jarring experience of having one's clinical competence called into question by a hospital's peer review process or by a licensing board. All of these potential sources of increased stress in the life of a physician can drain the coping reservoir and lead to further distress and/or maladaptive coping.

2. *Anxiety or Internal Conflict*: The experience of doubt or conflicting emotions about aspects of life and one's own decisions is commonplace, germane to a normal neurotic personality structure, and essential to a self-reflective process—important in the practice of medicine. However, if doubt and worry grow into excessive, pathological anxiety, the effect of the anxiety itself can be an extreme drain on fuel/energy. (Ironically, excessive worrying is rarely recognized as such by the worrier, perhaps due to the tendency to focus on the perceived problem.) Some physicians may question their choice of specialty or commitment to medicine. If distress deepens, a snowballing process may occur whereby symptoms of anxiety and depression can lead the individual to conclude that medicine or one's choice of specialty were wrong decisions. Reasoning based on negative emotions can result in distorted perceptions and a downward spiral leading to poor performance and worsening depression. Another source of internal conflict comes in the form of the keeping of a personal secret, such as a physician who has made a major medical error, but not acted in accordance with his or her conscience or ethical guidelines, or a gay medical student who has not come out yet to family or community. These secrets tend to weigh heavily as invisible sources of stress, which, when processed and worked through with a mentor or therapist, can lead to the release of an enormous emotional burden.

3. *Demands on time and energy*: There is probably not a single academic physician who has not experienced the challenge of juggling many responsibilities in a finite amount of time: professional responsibilities (clinical, administrative, and/or academic), family, partner, household, friends, and self (e.g., exercise, relaxation/recreation, spiritual practice). Over time, these demands, coupled with fatigue and guilt over unmet obligations can result

in burnout, which is characterized by three criteria: emotional exhaustion ("just going through the motions"); a diminished sense of achievement; and depersonalization (sense of detachment). While time is certainly a finite commodity, and energy may seem to fall into the same category, the energy that fuels resilience can be proactively monitored and replenished. Physicians can learn how to prevent the phenomenon of "running on empty" by understanding the signs of depletion, ideally learning to see it coming in advance and modifying accordingly, and knowing which activities provide the highest level of replenishment. In this way and counter to the prevailing societal view that "life happens to you," individuals can actually exert a reasonable level of control over the outcome of one's own well-being.

Replenishing Factors (Positive Inputs)

Some activities are essential to the basic human needs for rest and replenishment: sleep, good nutrition, and exercise. Perhaps surprisingly though, physicians and students who have high levels of clinical and scientific knowledge to apply to patient care and other professional activities, often need reminders that their own health will be negatively impacted if they shortchange sleep, healthy food, or exercise for long. Other potentially high-impact replenishing factors are included below.

1. *Psychosocial support*: Support can come from many sources within and outside the profession: spouse/partner, family, friends, peers/colleagues, and spiritual support. Psychosocial support can be more formal and provided by counselors, psychotherapists, or executive coaches. Specific groups, such as regional or local professional associations, can provide important support and practical information about how to balance the multiple demands of professional life.
2. *Mentoring*: Mentoring should not stop with the completion of medical training. Of the many important roles mentors fulfill, among the most vital are role modeling and supporting the art of balancing many roles, and recognizing the need for rest and

replenishing one's own reservoir. The ideal situation at any given time is to have a mentor or more likely, mentors, who can advise and consult on a regular or as needed basis, and also to be a mentor to more junior colleagues or trainees.

3. *Experiencing meaning and purpose*: Hard work and fatigue are far more satisfying and positive when they come as a result of investing oneself in something the practitioner finds meaningful and interesting. One challenge is to figure out which activities bring the greatest sense of meaning and purpose. For some physicians, a moment of connection or the act of helping a patient or student are extremely meaningful; for others, building or improving a healthcare system brings a greater sense of purpose. Self-awareness of which activities provide the greatest sense of wholeness, in professional or personal life, does not necessarily come automatically or completely intuitively but, rather, benefits from introspection and an attempt to objectively be a student of oneself and one's own life. How has it worked in the past? The experiences that had the highest emotional impact or clarified a particular career direction are probably still the types of activities that would serve as fuel for optimal coping in the present day. For many in academic medicine, the "meaning" of medicine is amplified through work as a clinician or teacher. Additionally, the arts and humanities significantly enhance life, and more specifically, advancing knowledge in the history of medicine or bioethics can be especially rewarding.

The Nature of the Coping Reservoir

The coping reservoir, like all human systems, is dynamic: ebbing and flowing, rising and falling over time. The goal is to keep the reservoir replenished. Given the burdens placed upon physicians and the inherent variability of individuals' resilience, it is probably unreasonable to expect the reservoir to be continuously full, brimming with high-octane fuel. Still, we must strive to keep the reservoir full *enough*.

Failure to keep the coping reservoir full enough can lead to cynicism, pessimism, frustration, burnout, and, eventually, depression.

While the topic of suicide prevention in physicians warrants much greater focus, the prevention of depression and recognition and treatment of symptoms of depression are known to be the best ways to prevent suicide. By finding ways to most effectively replenish the coping reservoir, resilience can flourish and, to the degree that is possible, suffering and disability can be prevented.

How to Keep the Reservoir Full (Enough)

Might it be possible to increase well-being, to diminish dysphoria, to feel more whole and present in the moment? And in a dynamic way over time, is it possible to adjust the positive and negative inputs to prevent burnout or crisis and optimize overall flourishing? If so, without necessarily changing the external circumstances of one's life, can an individual impact these outcomes? It *is* possible, even in the life of a physician, which tends to be tilted heavily in the direction of professional time and energy demands.

A proactive approach to keeping one's coping reservoir full is optimal if not required. Left unattended, most will find that as a matter of time and life's natural demands, the reservoir will drain, and the experience of running on empty leads to real consequences. Proactive approaches include the following:

1. Use a calendar as a tool to proactively plan healthy activities. While simple, scheduling health-promoting "nonnegotiables," e.g., sleep, exercise, quality time for important relationships, other high-impact activity outside of medicine, may allow professional demands and scheduling to be more balanced.
2. Have an inner circle of 1–3 trusted individuals with whom you can safely disclose concerns, e.g., partner, friend, mentor, colleague, therapist, pastor.
3. Establish care with a physician if you don't have one.
4. Pay attention to red flags: irritability and losing one's temper are often the first signs of imbalance; short-term memory slips are another sign of increased stress. Big red flags include increasing alcohol consumption or self-prescribing.
5. Take at least one real vacation each year.

6. Develop a list of priorities. This can be used to shape your decisions about how to approach which activities/relationships can be diminished versus increased. After creating your list, you may realize that a particular activity is actually lower on the list than it used to be, e.g., research or a relationship, and the acknowledgement of that change or revelation of an erroneous assumption may be instructive, allowing you to spend less time doing, or even take out, an activity.
7. Embrace the truth that you don't have to do and be everything at all times. In other words, career and life have natural phases, and with each changing phase, you can decide which set of roles is most important, appropriate, and feasible.
8. Be as compassionate with yourself as you would be with a loved one. This includes forgiving and being gracious with your own mistakes and shortcomings.

Conclusion

An important challenge to each physician and trainee is to be as serious a student of oneself as she/he is in other aspects of professional training. Most individuals are not inherently aware of the sources of "high-octane fuel" for their coping reservoir, and many assume that the drains are immutable. The knowledge and implementation of the regular practice of one's best replenishing input sources and diminishing the drains on one's coping reservoir requires a process of reflection, awareness, planning, and intention.

Examples of Positive Inputs
• Right amount of sleep on a regular basis
• Favorite types of exercise, e.g., running, yoga, dance, martial arts
• Mentoring trainees and witnessing their growth
• Connection and support from loved ones
• Processing conflict/challenging situation with mentor or trusted peer

- Other meaningful activities outside of medicine, e.g., arts, music, theater, literature
- Seeing your work make a difference
- Humor
- Flexible approach to problems
- Getting consultation on a difficult patient case
- Psychotherapy

Examples of Negative Inputs
- Anxiety that doesn't lead to a solution-oriented plan
- Fatigue especially if not addressed promptly
- Problematic, conflictual personal relationship
- Excess alcohol
- Sense of incompetence
- Sense of victimization by schedule, patient demands, flawed system
- Feeling rushed in patient care, decision-making
- Lack of connection with patients
- Secret keeping (not patient-related)
- Maintaining rigid approach to problems
- Being unwilling to admit vulnerability and imperfection

Words to the Wise
- Schedule health-promoting activities outside of medicine.
- Have an inner circle of trusted individuals with whom you can safely disclose concerns.
- Beware of irritability and losing your temper, which are often the first signs of imbalance, as well as short-term memory slips, increasing alcohol consumption, and self-prescribing.
- Embrace the truth that you do not have to do and be everything at all times.
- Be as compassionate with yourself as you would be with a loved one.

Ask Your Mentor or Colleagues

- What activity or part of life brings me the most sense of fulfillment? Can I reasonably increase the regularity or frequency of that activity? Conversely, which areas (people, activities) are the most draining?
- Are there problem/draining areas in my life that can be modified? Some things can't be removed from life completely, but can be modified. For example, a demanding administrative role you took on last year has become increasingly challenging and certain parts may be outside your areas of strength/expertise; are there any aspects that can be delegated or are actually not truly encompassed by that role? Another example: a demanding relative is part of your life, but you decide that it is possible to limit the amount or frequency of time spent with that person.
- Examine motivation: Am I doing certain activities because they seem important for academic promotion or to my mentors? Do I allow a conflictual relationship to continue because it is in fact a high-priority relationship, or out of a sense of helplessness or obligation? If it is a high-priority relationship, are there areas that could be improved via communication?

References

1. Wallace JE, Lemaire JB, Ghali WA. Physician wellness: a missing quality indicator. Lancet. 2009;374(9702):1714–21.
2. Scheurer D, McKean S, Miller J, Wetterneck T. U.S. physician satisfaction: a systematic review. J Hosp Med. 2009;4(9):560–8.
3. West CP, Huschka MM, Novotny PJ, Sloan JA, Kolars JC, Habermann TM, Shanafelt TD. Association of perceived medical errors with resident distress and empathy: a prospective longitudinal study. JAMA. 2006; 296(9):1071–8.
4. Dyrbye LN, Massie FS, Eacker A, Harper W, Power D, Durning SJ, Thomas MR, Moutier C, Satele D, Sloan JA, Shanafelt TD. Relationship between burnout and professional conduct and attitudes among US medical students: a Multi-Institutional Study. JAMA. 2010;304(11):1173–80.

5. Dyrbye LN, Thomas MR, Massie FS, Power DV, Eacker A, Harper W, Durning S, Moutier C, Szydlo DW, Novotny PJ, Sloan JA, Shanafelt TD. Burnout and suicidal ideation among US medical students. Ann Intern Med. 2008;149:334–41.
6. Schernhammer E. Taking their own lives- the high rate of physician suicide. N Eng J Med. 2005;352(24):2473–6.
7. Dunn LB, Iglewicz A, Moutier C. A conceptual model of medical student well-being: promoting resilience and preventing burnout. Acad Psychiatry. 2008;32(1):44–53.

How to Care for the Basics: Sleep, Nutrition, Exercise, Health

5

Christopher Guest and Rebecca Smith-Coggins

> *The best doctors in the world are Doctor Diet, Doctor Quiet, and Doctor Merryman.*
>
> Jonathan Swift

Balancing the demands of a life in academic medicine provides a unique challenge. We often find ourselves concentrating our efforts and energy on directly measurable outcomes like grants and tenure. Interestingly, we often neglect some of the most important factors sustaining our efforts. Faculty members are a driven group accustomed to sacrificing sleep, food, and physical activity to achieve their goals. Everyone can recall pulling the "all-nighter" before a big exam, usually accompanied by high calorie snacks and lots of coffee. This tradition reinvented itself in residency despite duty hour suggestions. Unfortunately, the tradition continues with manuscript deadlines and grant proposals. Paradoxically,

C. Guest, M.D., Ph.D. (✉)
Department of Emergency Medicine, Stanford University Hospital, 300 Pasteur Drive, Stanford, CA, USA
e-mail: cguest@stanford.edu

© Springer International Publishing Switzerland 2016
L.W. Roberts (ed.), *The Associate Professor Guidebook*,
DOI 10.1007/978-3-319-28001-1_5

by doing this we may be undermining our own efforts. A balanced diet, ample sleep, and physical activity are essential for peak performance. These three fundamental needs are not independent entities but interconnected and interactive. Historically, we have understood this on an intuitive level, but recent advances in molecular biology and psychoneuroimmunology have begun to elucidate the mechanistic principles guiding these interactions. With proper understanding of a few principles it is possible to utilize these interactions to form positive feedback loops which reinforce each other rather than detracting from one another. Additionally, these findings provide quantitative measures to guide our qualitative relationship to food, sleep, and exercise.

In this chapter we will discuss the importance of sleep, nutrition, and physical activity for optimal performance for academic faculty members. Each section will focus on the impact on overall health, metabolism, neuroimmune function, and tips for improving performance.

Sleep

A condition of body and mind such as that which typically recurs for several hours every night, in which the nervous system is relatively inactive, the eyes closed, the postural muscles relaxed, and consciousness practically suspended.

Oxford English Dictionary

During the last 30 years there has been an explosion of research into sleep. The drive for sleep is regulated by two processes. The first is a homeostatic process that dictates that the longer a person stays awake, the more a person needs to sleep. This process is coupled with our natural circadian rhythms, which set our natural threshold for initiating sleep or terminating it [1]. Another interesting finding is that although all humans have a requirement for sleep, the amount of sleep needed for optimal health varies from person to person and throughout the course of one's lifetime [2].

One of the fundamental elements of this research [3] has been to define sleep. With the invention of the electroencephalogram,

Alfred Loomis was able to define several distinct stages of sleep [4]. One of the widely accepted paradigms for defining sleep comes from the American Academy of Sleep Medicine (AASM), and it divides sleep into a slow wave component with three phases and a rapid wave state characterized by rapid eye movements (REM). The ratio of these phases changes over one's lifespan [3].

Sleep Patterns

Sleep patterns vary according to climate and local customs. In the USA, people typically work during the day and sleep at night. In climates with warm weather, it is not uncommon to take a midday nap lasting a few hours. This Mediterranean model takes advantage of the natural dip in alertness that is part of the circadian rhythm. The nature of our work has also changed with the shift away from a largely agrarian society with a heavy demand on physical labor to one that is predominantly based on providing services and manipulating and interpreting information. One factor that has greatly influenced our sleep cycle is the availability of cheap and reliable electricity. Not only does electricity allow us to extend the number of hours we work, but it also provides us with numerous other distractions like TV, computers, digital music players, and video games. Recent studies have shown that over the past 50 years the average duration of sleep per night has decreased by 1.5–2 h [5]. Several studies have been conducted in the USA to examine sleeping patterns during the last 50 years. A recent survey conducted by Gallup found that the average sleep duration was 6.8 h on weekdays and 7.4 h on weekends [3]. Two of the largest were surveys conducted by the American Cancer Society. One of the surveys done in 1959–1960 of more than a million Americans found that only 2 % of those surveyed reported sleeping less than 6 h per night. Interestingly a follow-up survey conducted in 1982 showed that nearly 20 % of adults reported sleeping less than 6 h [6]. An additional challenge that many physicians and scientists have to contend with is working shifts that do not coincide with our natural patterns of sleep and have been found to be associated with obesity, diabetes, and CVD [7]. Sleep deprivation can be categorized into acute and chronic. Acute deprivation is generally studied in people who have been awake for 24–72 h. This type of deprivation can have profound and dangerous effects including hallucinations and psychosis [8]. Chronic deprivation is characterized by limiting the amount of sleep a person gets each night over a period of time, usually around 4–6 h. This type of sleep deprivation is a more accurate representation of what we are more likely to encounter in our daily lives. With chronic sleep deprivation a number of interesting phenomena occur. Not only are there metabolic, immune, and cognitive changes, but the person's perception of his or her deficits also change [9]. These changes vary from person to person and with the degree of sleep deprivation but are generally well conserved within the same person, much like a personality trait [10]. Additionally, with chronic sleep deprivation a sleep debt builds up over time, and the debt can act like an episode of acute sleep deprivation if it goes on long enough [11]. Fortunately, this debt can be paid back by getting extra sleep.

Why Is Sleep Important?

One of the most powerful observations about sleep from an evolutionary perspective is that all mammals must sleep. Although we do not fully understand why, there must be a substantial survival benefit to sleep. Indeed, there have been a number of studies that look at the relationship of sleep duration on survival, and they have found that sleep duration of less than 7 h is associated with an increased mortality risk [12, 13]. Interestingly, this relationship is not linear. The benefit begins to decrease as sleep duration exceeds 8.5 h, and increased sleep is actually associated with a higher mortality. Additionally, this finding is also mirrored when analyzing coronary heart disease [14]. One study showed that when sleep is limited to less than 5 h per night, subjects were 2–3 times more likely to have an adverse cardiovascular event [15]. This area is actively being investigated, and interesting metabolic and immune alterations found in the sleep deprived are likely culprits; however, establishing a causal relationship is difficult, given the multitude of factors at work [16]. These general findings are disturbing but offer potential opportunities for interventions.

In addition to the general increased risk of mortality and cardiovascular disease, recent evidence also has shown a role for sleep as key modifier of endocrine and immune function. Sleep restriction has been shown to have a number of deleterious effects on glucose tolerance, activation of the sympathetic nervous system, and thyrotropin. Additionally, decreased sleep is associated with an increase in obesity and dysregulation of two important hormones that regulate appetite and satiety. These changes are also associated with an increase in proinflammatory cytokines [17], which have been shown to increase insulin resistance [18]. These proinflammatory cytokines have been shown to increase depressive-like behavior and reduce social activity [19]. Taken together, this evidence suggests an important role for sleep and the regulation of our endocrine function.

Along with the physiological changes found with sleep deprivation, another important impact of sleep deprivation is a decrease in cognitive performance. Although acute sleep deprivation has been more thoroughly studied, chronic sleep deprivation is more applicable to our daily lives and will be focused on here. Sleep deprivation has been shown to have deleterious effects on working memory, long-term memory, attention, and decision making [20]. Many of the changes in cognition found with sleep deprivation can be ascribed to decreased attention or vigilance. This decreased attention has a cascade function, decreasing one's ability to integrate new information and respond appropriately to a variety of stimuli and tasks. Additionally, recent work has shown that sleep-deprived people actually periodically undergo moments of microsleep, which can last anywhere from a fraction of a second to 10 s in duration [21]. As one can imagine, these events are especially dangerous when driving, operating heavy machinery, or conducting any other tasks where irreversible mistakes can easily be made. Interestingly, as sleep deprivation increases, one's insight of performance becomes worse [22]. These effects have been shown with chronic sleep deprivation of less than 7 h per night and increase as the sleep interval decreases [3]. Fortunately, brief naps of only 10 min have been shown to significantly improve alertness and performance [23] and may play an important role for restoring function to appropriate levels for individuals with demanding lifestyles subject to chronic sleep deprivation.

Getting the Most from Sleep

Adequate Time

Perhaps one of the most obvious and difficult variables to control for getting the most from sleep is finding adequate time. Research has shown that physicians are more likely than the general population to be sleep deprived, which can contribute to poor outcomes for our patients and for our well-being [24]. One way to help alleviate this shortage is to view adequate sleep as a necessity like food, water, or air and make it a priority that is not subject to cuts. There are always going to be occasions when we have to shave a little time off our regular sleep schedule, but it should not become common, and the sleep debt should be repaid as quickly as possible to ensure peak performance. The amount of time one needs varies from individual to individual; however, most studies indicate that performance, satisfaction, and overall wellness are higher with between 6.5 and 9 h of sleep [3].

Sleep Hygiene

A number of components contribute to sleep hygiene. One way to understand sleep hygiene is to break it into two components—environmental and non-environmental. The environmental factors include comfortable bedding and a dark, cool, and quite space dedicated to sleep. The space should not include a TV or digital distractions. For shift workers black-out curtains are important so that alterations in the influence of the circadian rhythm can be minimized. Some people even find it useful to use artificial light sources to initiate the waking part of the sleep cycle. White noise can be provided by a fan or a white noise machine or earplugs can be used.

Non-environmental factors include exercise, diet, pharmacological agents like sleep aids and stimulants like caffeine. Exercise can be an important sleep aid if timed correctly. Exercise can act to reduce muscular tension that builds throughout a stressful day. This muscular tension can contribute to less restful sleep. Additionally, exercise can have an anxiolytic effect [25], reducing yet another non-environmental factor contributing to poor sleep.

Rigorous exercise should be avoided about 2 h before sleep in order to allow the stimulation of the exercise to wane and the body to fully relax. Similarly, eating a light snack may aid in sleep while having a large meal within 4 h may cause sleep disturbances [26]. Additionally, there are many pharmacological agents that can affect sleep. Two of the most common are alcohol and caffeine. Initially, alcohol has a sedative effect and promotes sleep initiation; however, alcohol use can cause disruption to our natural sleep cycle and can change the proportion of slow wave sleep [27]. Caffeine can plan an important role of promoting attention and vigilance even while sleep deprived [28] but there is a difficult balance that must be struck in order to ensure that we are still able to achieve adequate and restful sleep after using caffeine [29]. Abstaining from caffeine for 4 h prior to sleep is prudent to avoid some of the sleep disruptions found by using caffeine to increase wakefulness [30]. Some other popular sleep aids include diphenhydramine and melatonin. Diphenhydramine is thought to act by antagonizing the histamine and its alertness-promoting properties. Unfortunately, diphenhydramine has a number of side effects and limited efficacy. Newer prescription medications include zolpidem and zaleplon. These medications are thought to have fewer side effects but some of their unique side effects include sleep eating [31, 32]. Interestingly, melatonin is an endogenous hormone produced by the pineal gland that is an important regulator of the sleep–wake cycle. Melatonin has been shown to help with some sleep disorders [33]. It does not have the same potential for

Dos and Do Nots of Good Sleep Hygiene

Do	Do not
Limit screen time within 2 h of bedtime	Keep a TV in your room
Sleep in a dark room	Drink caffeine within 4 h of bedtime
Sleep in a cool room	Exercise an hour before sleep time
Sleep in a quiet environment	Drink too much alcohol
Use some white noise like a fan	
Take a warm bath 30 min before sleep	

habituation and it works to normalize internal circadian drives rather than to suppress alertness like other sleep aids.

Sleep Summary

Sleep has held a place of mystery and reverence for humankind. The ancient Greeks believed that our sleeping life was an important time for rejuvenation and revelations from the gods. The purpose of sleep is still largely a mystery. Some evidence suggests that it is important for wound healing. Animals subjected to sleep deprivation have shown substantial healing deficits when compared to controls. Additionally, sleep provides an opportunity for energy conservation, decreasing energy demands by 5–15 %. Interestingly energy conservation does not seem to be the chief benefit of sleep. Hibernating animals will periodically shift from a low energy state into a higher energy demand sleep to fulfill some other vital function [34]. Sleep is also an important regulator of endocrine, immune, and cognitive function. As physicians we face unique challenges to maintaining a healthy balance between sleep and the rest of our activities, but we are now different than others in our absolute need for sleep. Sleep must remain a priority for us in order to ensure our optimal health and the safety of our patients.

Nutrition and Physical Activity

> *If we could give every individual the right amount of nourishment and exercise, not too little and not too much, we would have found the safest way to health.*

> Hippocrates

Nutritional Balance: Body Composition as an Indicator of Health

We often think of nutrition as a dirty word. It can make us feel guilty for the food choices we have made or are going to make. But, like other health components, the most important thing in diet is balance. One way to assess dietary balance in an individual is by evaluating body composition. Body composition is often more meaningful than simply measuring weight or using Body Mass Index (BMI) values because it provides more individualized information. Simply put, body composition can be divided into three components: fat, bone, and muscle mass; which provide an easy-to-use framework to evaluate general health or risk for chronic diseases.

The fat mass component of body composition is an important and complicated one. Adipose is metabolically active and key for storage of lipid-soluble vitamins and energy as well as healthy production of an array of hormones, among other functions. On the other hand excessive fat, which may be uncomfortable or unsightly, is also unhealthy for a number of reasons. Extra weight puts additional strain and stress on joints and pressure on internal organs. Adipose around the mid-section has been linked to increased risk for a number of diseases including cardiovascular disease, pre-diabetes, and diabetes [35, 36]. Additionally, high adiposity increases risk for sleep apnea disrupting sleep and adding a number of health risk factors associated with sleep deprivation.

It is well established that adults reach their peak muscle and bone mass by the fourth decade of life (or their early 30s) [37, 38]. As a result, it is of utmost importance to spend the teen and young adult years building a solid foundation in regard to these composites. Additionally it is important to establish good habits in these formative years, so that upon middle age one can continue to mitigate these losses. Reduction in skeletal muscle mass can be associated with declines in strength, endurance, and muscle power. Reduction in bone mass tends to be a slower process that can be even more devastating to overall health and function later in life.

Strategies for Adults to Obtain a Healthy Body Composition

Healthy body composition at any age is influenced by three main factors: hormones, nutrition, and physical activity. Hormones remain fairly steady through young adulthood and middle age, with a major exceptions being pregnancy and lactation—which is beyond the scope of this chapter. For this reason we will focus on nutrition and physical activity.

Nutrition

Nutrition is a relatively young science that, like sleep, is actively being studied. Because it affects all people there are a number of bodies that govern the study and supply of food in the USA. These groups include the Food and Nutrition Board (FNB) of the Institute of Medicine (IOM), The Department of Health and Human Services (HHS), and the US Department of Agriculture (USDA). They are responsible for nutrition recommendations and have established nutrient intake recommendations across the lifespan. For the purposes of these recommendations, the dietary plans are divided by calorie level (which is variable depending on individual needs). These recommendations are further divided into food groups within calorie levels for both men (average calorie range: 1800–2600) and women (average calorie range: 1400–2200) to ensure meeting various nutrient needs [39]. It is important to note that these recommendations are for healthy adults. For those with specific nutritional needs (e.g., people who take certain medications, those with diabetes) consultation with a registered dietitian would be most appropriate to receive specific diet advice.

Energy (Calorie) Needs

Calorie needs remain fairly steady following adolescence through middle age. Most important is matching energy intake with energy expenditure. As expected, the more active a person is, the higher caloric needs will be—at any stage of life. It is important to balance nutrients (carbohydrate, protein, fat, vitamins, and minerals) within the appropriate calorie level and focus on nutrient dense foods (high nutrients/g) to ensure maximal health and weight management [39].

Carbohydrates

Carbohydrate sources include grains (rice, breads, pasta, etc.), fruits, and some vegetables. In mid-life and older adults insulin resistance may start to become an issue, leading to people becoming "carb-conscious." While balancing carbohydrate intake with insulin is important, it is not generally recommended that people eliminate carbohydrates from their diet under normal circumstances because of their use by the body (and especially the brain) as fuel. Nor is it necessary to increase carbohydrate intake in relation to the rest of the diet [39]. An important subgroup of carbohydrates is fiber. Fiber is important for maintaining proper stomach and intestinal health (e.g., providing nourishment to some of the cells that line the gut as well as preventing constipation) and higher intakes have been associated with lower incidence of colon cancer and lower levels of circulating cholesterol as well as for triggering feelings of fullness [40].

Fats

Dietary fat (lipids) is also a key element as it not only provides flavor and texture to foods but also carries fat-soluble vitamins, acts as an important building block for many hormones, and performs other essential functions throughout the body. Fat does not make a person fat. However, excessive intake of fat (more than 30 % of calories from fat), which is calorically-dense, can contribute to obesity. Not all fats are created equal. It is important to focus on higher intake of the healthy fats: mono-unsaturated fatty acids (MUFAs; olive oil, avocados, etc.), poly-unsaturated fatty acids (PUFAs; nuts, seeds, etc.) and specifically omega-3 and -6 oils (found in fatty fish and nuts) and lower intake of saturated fats (found in red meat, butter, etc.) and trans-fats (found in processed foods like shortening and pre-packaged crackers, cookies, etc.).

Protein

Protein is the key macronutrient for muscle building and maintenance. The mantra of many dietitians when it comes to protein is "lean, high-quality protein." Sources like fish, poultry (skin removed), dairy (low or no fat), and soy should be a major focus in the diet because they provide the nourishment without the added calories of fat. There is evidence that high protein meals increase feelings of fullness without the feelings of sluggishness that fatty meals provide. However, moderation is important here too. While protein provides many benefits, like the other macronutrients, too much can result in weight gain.

Weight Management

Generally, it is recommended that healthy adults maintain a BMI of 18–24.9. Interestingly, a BMI under 18 is associated with an increased mortality while a BMI of 25–29.9 was found to be associated with a decrease in noncancer and noncardiac death. As expected an elevated BMI is associated with increased cardiac mortality [41]. Preventing weight gain is much easier than losing weight, but in this age of calorically dense, easy-to-get food, it is often easier said than done. The primary approach is to achieve a sustainable healthy lifestyle that includes a varied diet and plenty of physical activity.

Consuming fewer calories through dietary changes appears to promote weight loss more effectively than does exercise and physical activity. But physical activity is also important in weight control. The key to weight loss is burning more calories than are consumed. Exercise plus calorie restriction can help provide the weight-loss edge. Exercise can help burn off the excess calories one cannot cut through diet alone. Exercise also offers numerous health benefits, including boosting mood, strengthening the cardiovascular system, and reducing blood pressure.

Exercise can also help in *maintaining* weight loss. Studies show that people who maintain their weight loss over the long term get regular physical activity [42]. In contrast, people who lose weight by crash dieting or by drastically reducing their calories to 400–800 a day are likely to regain weight quickly, often within 6 months after they stop dieting. If there is a great amount of weight to be lost, the expertise of a registered dietitian may be needed to provide appropriate nutritional counseling.

Weight loss calculation: Because 3500 cal equals about 1 lb (0.45 kg) of fat, one needs to burn 3500 cal more than one takes in to lose 1 lb. So if one cuts 500 cal from his or her typical diet each day, one would lose about 1 lb a week (500 cal×7 days = 3500 cal).

Physical Activity

Regarding maintenance of general health, energy, stamina, and a proportional body composition, physical activity is just as important as a balanced diet. Physical *inactivity* is directly linked to reduced muscle mass and quality and associated reductions in physical functional ability, and habitual physical activity has been consistently associated with improvements in physical function [43]. The four main guidelines for activity are: (1) avoid inactivity; (2) substantial health benefits can be gained from medium amounts of aerobic activity; (3) more health benefits can be gained from high amounts of aerobic activity; and (4) muscle-strengthening activities provide additional health benefits.

Current exercise recommendations are based on levels where substantial health benefits are achieved. For these benefits, each week adults should do at least 150 min of moderate-intensity aerobic physical activity or 75 min of vigorous-intensity aerobic activity or an equivalent combination of moderate- and vigorous-intensity aerobic activity. Ideally, this activity is performed in episodes of at least 10 min and preferably spread throughout the week [44].

For young and middle-aged adults, a well-rounded exercise program will include training for muscle strength, endurance, and power. Additionally, programs that include flexibility and balance training are important to include for maximal functionality throughout the lifespan.

In addition to the "physical" benefits of exercise for function, it is important to recognize the psychological aspects as well. Reduced muscle mass and strength decreases the capacity to perform physical work and the relative workload of a given task and increases fatigue. An adult who is more physically active will find that fatigue can be reduced.

How to Meet These Guidelines Easily Throughout the Week

Take a brisk 10-min walk two times a day. This can include a walk outside, a walk to the car (parked a little farther away), or taking the stairs instead of the elevator—anything that elevates the heart rate for 10 min at a time. However one decides to spend those walks each day, these bouts add up to 120 min. To get that additional 30 min, try playing with kids or pets outside two to three times each week, or add three 10 min walks. Another way to meet or exceed these guidelines is to take 15-min walks instead.

Too hard to keep track of all those 10-min bouts? Become a weekend warrior! Physical activity guidelines were adjusted a few years back because there was evidence that even if one meets these guidelines in a single timeframe, health benefits were still achieved. This may actually work better for the busy schedule of a physician. The point is to stay active.

How do you tell the difference between "moderate" and "vigorous" activity? Take the *Talk Test*. Can you still carry on a conversation but not sing—your activity is moderate. Can't get more than a couple words out? That's vigorous activity!

Nutrition and Physical Activity Summary

This section highlighted the importance of physical activity and nutrition behaviors to maintain the health of the three main components of body composition (fat, bone, and lean mass), in adults. Good nutrition and physical activity practices are of primary importance in overall health and well-being. Additionally, a healthy body composition can also enhance psychological well-being, by providing improvements in sleep, self esteem, and productivity at work and at home as well as reductions in anxiety and stress.

Consulting with nutrition and exercise experts is essential when attempting changes with regard to physical activity and nutrition behaviors, particularly if you are unfamiliar with how to get started with a healthy lifestyle. The human body remains remarkably adaptable to change even well into old age, and it is never too early or too late to experience the physical and psychological benefits of healthy lifestyle choices.

Conclusion

You cannot take care of other people if you do not take care of yourself. Ample sleep, a balanced diet, and physical activity are three fundamental needs. They are not independent entities, but interconnected and interactive.

Words to the Wise
- View adequate sleep as a necessity like food, water, or air, and make it a priority that is not subject to cuts.
- The most important thing in diet is balance.
- Exercise may be easier to fit in using 10-min increments throughout the day or longer weekend sessions to total 120 min.

Ask Your Mentor or Colleagues
- How do you find the time to eat well and/or exercise regularly?
- How do you recommend I manage my time?

References

1. Achermann P. The two-process model of sleep regulation revisited. Aviat Space Environ Med. 2004;75(3 Suppl):A37–43.
2. Dinges DF. Sleep debt and scientific evidence. Sleep. 2004;27(6): 1050–2.
3. Banks S, Dinges DF. Behavioral and physiological consequences of sleep restriction. J Clin Sleep Med. 2007;3(5):519–28.

4. Davis H, Davis PA, et al. Changes in human brain potentials during the onset of sleep. Science. 1937;86(2237):448–50.

5. Knutson KL, Van Cauter E, et al. Trends in the prevalence of short sleepers in the USA: 1975–2006. Sleep. 2010;33(1):37–45.

6. Van Cauter E, Knutson KL. Sleep and the epidemic of obesity in children and adults. Eur J Endocrinol. 2008;159 Suppl 1:S59–66.

7. Pedrosa RP, Lima SG, et al. Sleep quality and quality of life in patients with hypertrophic cardiomyopathy. Cardiology. 2010;117(3):200–6.

8. Yoo SS, Gujar N, et al. The human emotional brain without sleep–a prefrontal amygdala disconnect. Curr Biol. 2007;17(20):R877–8.

9. Van Dongen HP, Maislin G, et al. The cumulative cost of additional wakefulness: dose-response effects on neurobehavioral functions and sleep physiology from chronic sleep restriction and total sleep deprivation. Sleep. 2003;26(2):117–26.

10. Van Dongen HP, Baynard MD, et al. Systematic interindividual differences in neurobehavioral impairment from sleep loss: evidence of trait-like differential vulnerability. Sleep. 2004;27(3):423–33.

11. Belenky G, Wesensten NJ, et al. Patterns of performance degradation and restoration during sleep restriction and subsequent recovery: a sleep dose-response study. J Sleep Res. 2003;12(1):1–12.

12. Tamakoshi A, Ohno Y. Self-reported sleep duration as a predictor of all-cause mortality: results from the JACC study, Japan. Sleep. 2004;27(1): 51–4.

13. Ferrie JE, Shipley MJ, et al. A prospective study of change in sleep duration: associations with mortality in the Whitehall II cohort. Sleep. 2007;30(12):1659–66.

14. Ayas NT, White DP, et al. A prospective study of sleep duration and coronary heart disease in women. Arch Intern Med. 2003;163(2):205–9.

15. Liu Y, Tanaka H. Overtime work, insufficient sleep, and risk of non-fatal acute myocardial infarction in Japanese men. Occup Environ Med. 2002;59(7):447–51.

16. Puttonen S, Harma M, et al. Shift work and cardiovascular disease - pathways from circadian stress to morbidity. Scand J Work Environ Health. 2010;36(2):96–108.

17. Irwin MR, Carrillo C, et al. Sleep loss activates cellular markers of inflammation: sex differences. Brain Behav Immun. 2010;24(1):53–7.

18. O'Connor JC, Sherry CL, et al. Type 2 diabetes impairs insulin receptor substrate-2-mediated phosphatidylinositol 3-kinase activity in primary macrophages to induce a state of cytokine resistance to IL-4 in association with overexpression of suppressor of cytokine signaling-3. J Immunol. 2007;178(11):6886–93.

19. Guest CB, Park MJ, et al. The implication of proinflammatory cytokines in type 2 diabetes. Front Biosci. 2008;13:5187–94.

20. Alhola P, Polo-Kantola P. Sleep deprivation: impact on cognitive performance. Neuropsychiatr Dis Treat. 2007;3(5):553–67.

21. Priest B, Brichard C, et al. Microsleep during a simplified maintenance of wakefulness test. A validation study of the OSLER test. Am J Respir Crit Care Med. 2001;163(7):1619–25.
22. Harrison Y, Horne JA. The impact of sleep deprivation on decision making: a review. J Exp Psychol Appl. 2000;6(3):236–49.
23. Tietzel AJ, Lack LC. The short-term benefits of brief and long naps following nocturnal sleep restriction. Sleep. 2001;24(3):293–300.
24. Olson EJ, Drage LA, et al. Sleep deprivation, physician performance, and patient safety. Chest. 2009;136(5):1389–96.
25. Vollert C, Zagaar M, et al. Exercise prevents sleep deprivation-associated anxiety-like behavior in rats: potential role of oxidative stress mechanisms. Behav Brain Res. 2011;224(2):233–40.
26. Barion A, Zee PC. A clinical approach to circadian rhythm sleep disorders. Sleep Med. 2007;8(6):566–77.
27. Landolt HP, Roth C, et al. Late-afternoon ethanol intake affects nocturnal sleep and the sleep EEG in middle-aged men. J Clin Psychopharmacol. 1996; 16(6):428–36.
28. Horne J, Reyner L. Vehicle accidents related to sleep: a review. Occup Environ Med. 1999;56(5):289–94.
29. Landolt HP, Retey JV, et al. Caffeine attenuates waking and sleep electroencephalographic markers of sleep homeostasis in humans. Neuropsychopharmacology. 2004;29(10):1933–9.
30. Snel J, Lorist MM. Effects of caffeine on sleep and cognition. Prog Brain Res. 2011;190:105–17.
31. Hoque R, Chesson Jr AL. Zolpidem-induced sleepwalking, sleep related eating disorder, and sleep-driving: fluorine-18-flourodeoxyglucose positron emission tomography analysis, and a literature review of other unexpected clinical effects of zolpidem. J Clin Sleep Med. 2009;5(5):471–6.
32. Ringdahl EN, Pereira SL, et al. Treatment of primary insomnia. J Am Board Fam Pract. 2004;17(3):212–9.
33. van Geijlswijk IM, Korzilius HP, et al. The use of exogenous melatonin in delayed sleep phase disorder: a meta-analysis. Sleep. 2010;33(12):1605–14.
34. Palchykova S, Deboer T, et al. Selective sleep deprivation after daily torpor in the Djungarian hamster. J Sleep Res. 2002;11(4):313–9.
35. Donahue RP, Abbott RD. Central obesity and coronary heart disease in men. Lancet. 1987;2(8569):1215.
36. Rexrode KM, Carey VJ, et al. Abdominal adiposity and coronary heart disease in women. JAMA. 1998;280(21):1843–8.
37. Bonjour JP, Theintz G, et al. Peak bone mass. Osteoporos Int. 1994;4 Suppl 1:7–13.
38. Ferretti G, Narici MV, et al. Determinants of peak muscle power: effects of age and physical conditioning. Eur J Appl Physiol Occup Physiol. 1994;68(2):111–5.
39. United States. Dept. of Health and Human Services, United States. Dept. of Agriculture, et al. Dietary guidelines for Americans, 2010. GPO: Washington, DC; 2010.

40. Bourdon I, Olson B, et al. Beans, as a source of dietary fiber, increase cholecystokinin and apolipoprotein b48 response to test meals in men. J Nutr. 2001;131(5): 1485–90.
41. Eckel RH, Krauss RM. American Heart Association call to action: obesity as a major risk factor for coronary heart disease. AHA Nutrition Committee. Circulation. 1998;97(21):2099–100.
42. Anderson JW, Konz EC, et al. Long-term weight-loss maintenance: a meta-analysis of US studies. Am J Clin Nutr. 2001;74(5):579–84.
43. Brach JS, Simonsick EM, et al. The association between physical function and lifestyle activity and exercise in the health, aging and body composition study. J Am Geriatr Soc. 2004;52(4):502–9.
44. Haskell WL, Lee IM, et al. Physical activity and public health: updated recommendation for adults from the American College of Sports Medicine and the American Heart Association. Med Sci Sports Exerc. 2007;39(8): 1423–34.

How to Manage Personal Finances

6

David J. Peterson and Roger Strode

For the academic faculty member, managing personal finances is as essential as the time, effort, and planning that were invested to acquire the educational credentials to support an academic appointment in medicine. After devoting years of study to achieve an M.D. or Ph.D. degree, and then more years in residency, fellowship or other postdoctoral learning programs, the academic faculty member needs to attend, with equal fervor, to his or her financial health in order to sustain the academic career and allow it to flourish. Simply stated, the academic faculty member's investment in education requires a return on that investment and this return can be measured in a variety of ways. Certainly an example of such a return is academic success evidenced through scholarly work, but an equally important return is also realized through a salary, benefits, and a myriad of other financial products that provide for his or her financial well-being throughout an academic career and extending through retirement.

Managing personal finances can be viewed as one component of taking care of "Me, Inc.," and in fact was characterized as such in a keynote address at an annual conference of medical group professionals [1]. "Me, Inc." goes beyond thinking of oneself in the

D.J. Peterson, M.B.A., F.A.C.M.P.E. (✉)
Department of Psychiatry and Behavioral Medicine,
Medical College of Wisconsin, 8701 Watertown Plank Road,
Milwaukee, WI, USA
e-mail: Peterson@mcw.edu

© Springer International Publishing Switzerland 2016
L.W. Roberts (ed.), *The Associate Professor Guidebook*,
DOI 10.1007/978-3-319-28001-1_6

financial context of a salary alone and extends to thinking of oneself as a business, a multifaceted business with a diverse set of intangible and tangible assets such as education, reputation, bank, and investment accounts, home and other household and material goods. "Me, Inc." also includes liabilities such as educational loans, home and auto loans, and other financial commitments such as credit card debt, to name a few. The difference between the academic household's financial assets and liabilities can be viewed as *net worth*, a number that will ideally grow to a large positive number that can sustain the faculty member throughout his or her life.

Just like managing any business, managing "Me, Inc." requires knowledge of some fundamental personal finance principles and products along with an ability to think in both the short and long term. It means financially planning for a "worst case" like death or disability, planning for both welcome and unwelcome health events, planning for financial surprises, planning for an eventual retirement, long-term care and eventually death, and certainly planning for all of the living that occurs in between.

Personal Finance Basics

Because the topic of personal finance touches everyone, everyone has an opinion and is often not afraid to share it. Name a "money" topic, and there will be a variety of opinions, opinions that can be confusing and conflicting. Need a car? Someone will state that it is better to lease versus buy, while an equally persuasive argument can be made for a purchase over a lease. Need a place to live? Conventional wisdom states that buying a home is a "good investment" but that is not always the case. Got some money to invest? Financial experts in the guise of investment advisors, money managers, financial planners and insurance salesmen—all with the perquisite credentials—will make equally compelling arguments in favor of stocks, bonds, real estate, precious metals, and insurance products, to name a few.

Fortunately, there are a few commonly-accepted demographic trends and principles in the financial world that can help guide the academic faculty member through the maze of products and options.

Demographically, data show that the general US population is living longer and is more active as it ages. For example, according to the Centers for Disease Control, the average life expectancy for an individual in 1980 was 73.88 years. In 2007 the average life expectancy grew to 77.9 years [2]. Along with living longer, senior citizens are more active, "pursuing freedom, not retirement" [3]. This trend of increasing longevity coupled with a more active lifestyle affects how much the academic family should save, how long the academic faculty member will work and what kind of lifestyle expectations can be afforded. "Saving more and working longer" are obvious answers, but even these answers are clearly dependent upon an individual's goals, expectations and health.

To ensure that a family has enough funds to support these trends, it helps to remember a principal principle in money and finance. The "*time value of money*" is a foundation principle stating that the value of money will change over time at varying interest rates. It can either go up or down, depending upon the interest rate and whether the money will be collected in the future or in the present. For example, $100 now growing at a 5 % simple interest rate will be worth $105 at the end of 12 months. This would be the *future value* of money. Conversely, the *present value* of $105 12 months into the future, discounted at the same interest rate, represents $100 now [4].

The time value of money is a financial principle that underlies the value of general savings accounts, certificates of deposit, stock and bond investments, it is used in house mortgage and other lease/buy calculations and is certainly a fundamental principle in calculating the value and cost of insurance products, for example. It is the concept that allows household savings to grow over time, sometimes to large amounts, even with small but steady contributions early in a career.

An example of how time affects the value of money, the "*Rule of 72*" (72/interest rate=years to double) is an easy way to calculate approximately how long it will take for a sum of money to double at any given interest rate [5]. For example, if an individual invests $1000 now at an interest rate of 6 %, the money will double to $2000 in approximately 12 years (72/6=12). At a 12 % interest rate that sum will grow to $2000 in approximately 6 years (72/12=6).

Financial experts will also point to other generally-accepted rules of thumb:

- The idea that some debt is "good," especially debt for a tangible asset that appreciates in value, such as a mortgage for a house. Conversely, some debt is "bad," with revolving debt, i.e., credit cards, as the prime example [6].
- A "pay yourself first" philosophy that essentially states that an individual or family—"Me, Inc.," for example—should stand first in line when paying bills each month. "Pay yourself first" usually means a contribution to a savings account or other investment account, just as one would pay another bill such as the phone, electricity, or gas bill. Automatic savings plans such as those with a payroll deduction or through an automatic, regular monthly withdrawal for a savings account is a classic way to execute this plan [7].
- A philosophy that "tax deferral and avoidance" is usually a good financial strategy. Tax evasion is clearly illegal, but tax avoidance and tax deferral are legitimate strategies to utilize when managing personal finances. A smart tax strategy makes assumptions though, assumptions such as future income (is it rising or falling?) or future federal and state tax policy (are rates rising or falling?). The answer to either might mean paying taxes now is a smarter strategy than deferring taxes into the next year where future income might be subject to either higher rates or a higher income tax bracket. Pre-tax payroll deductions and an effective use of flexible spending, health, or dependent accounts are also useful tools when deploying a tax-deferral/avoidance strategy. Saving for retirement through tax-deferred investment vehicles such as 401(k)s and 403(b)s is an ideal example of deploying such a tax and savings strategy.
- An opinion that fee-based financial advisors are preferable over advisors that earn their fee from commissions on the type of investment sold. As a general rule, fee-based advisors are considered more impartial and in theory offer unbiased investment advice because their fee is not based on the type of investment strategy used, such as that with advisors who make a commission on the type of investment chosen [8].

- A mantra of "diversify, diversify, diversify." Most everyone will agree that smart money management and "downside" risk management—in other words, "protecting the household net worth"—requires a diversification of investments over several financial products such as a house, insurance, cash and money market accounts, stocks and bonds, and other investment vehicles. The theory is, quite simply, that when one asset goes down, the other assets will retain their value or even increase, offsetting the loss in one asset. This notion was sorely tested in the world financial crisis that began in 2008, but diversification is still considered a prudent financial strategy [9].

Finally, most experts and advisors will agree that effective money management requires some level of professional expertise. Given the complexities and varieties of money management choices today, both the time to manage the household finances and the expertise to do so need to be available. Often there is a paucity of at least one, if not both, so when that is the case, identifying a trusted advisor—ideally fee-based as noted above—is a wise strategy.

Personal Income Management

During his or her working years, a cornerstone of annual income for "Me, Inc." will likely be the academic faculty member's *annual salary*, based on some type of pay scale established by the State (if a public institution) or by some other benchmark such as the Association of American Medical Colleges (AAMC). The baseline salary for the faculty member is often negotiated and established in the hiring process. Thereafter, changes in annual salary are often governed by the cost of living, merit, changes in rank, and years of service to name a few. In some instances, bonuses or other incentives may increase the annual salary.

In addition to an annual salary, a generally rich package of other *fringe benefits* usually accompanies an academic appointment. Benefits such as annual vacation, sick leave, and insurance coverage are standard. Insurance coverages usually include a major medical insurance package, dental insurance, life insurance and short and long-term disability coverage. Generous sick leave allowances are sometimes offered in lieu of short-term disability, but in any event, the faculty member should be protected in the case of an inability to work in either the short or the long-term.

A relatively new addition to the standard package of benefits is some form of "flexible spending account" (FSA) that allows the faculty member to shelter salary dollars on a pre-tax basis to support certain medical, dental and dependent expenses. What can be purchased or supported by these pre-tax dollars and how much can be sheltered are defined by federal tax and health care rules. Usually, there is a "use it or lose it" aspect to sheltering such dollars—that is, no carryover of unspent funds from year to year.

Health care savings accounts (HSAs) are also a newer pre-tax option for faculty. HSAs allow for sheltering salary dollars to pay for medical expense and these too are defined by law, but are often allowed to carryover from year to year.

The advantage to both FSAs and HSAs is the ability to shelter salary income from taxes for expenses that the faculty member would or could incur and normally would pay for with after-tax salary dollars. The savings can be significant. For example, a faculty member in a 30 % tax bracket can shelter $1000 in support of eligible expenses at a cost of only $700.

Finally, some type of eligibility for a retirement plan is a standard component of an annual salary and benefit package. There are two basic types of retirement plans, a *defined benefit* and *defined contribution* plan [10]. Defined benefit plans, offered by ever fewer employers, generally define a retirement benefit using a formula that is based on years of service to an organization. A simple defined benefit formula might be "years of service × 2 % for each year × the average of the last 3 years of salary." Using this formula, for example, a faculty member with 35 years of service and an average annual salary of $100,000 could expect annual retirement income totaling $70,000 ($35 \times 0.02 \times \$100,000$). There are a number of pros and cons attached to such plans. Some of the pros include simplicity and predictability while one con is the limited choice that such a plan offers along with the limited ability to change employers.

Defined contribution plans, on the other hand, define the contribution the organization is making toward the retirement plan, rather than the benefit. Such plans (usually defined and allowed under 401(k), 403(b) or 457(b) tax law) usually require the faculty member to contribute "*x*%" of his or her annual faculty salary, matched by an organizational contribution of "*X* %" of the faculty member's salary [10]. These funds are then regularly directed into a mutual fund account containing investment options (stocks, bonds, money market, real estate investment trusts, etc.) that will rise or fall with the economic climate. For example, a faculty member earning $100,000 annually might have a defined contribution plan that requires the faculty member to contribute 5 % of gross income that is then matched with a 10 % contribution by the organization, allowing a total of $15,000 annually to be contributed to a mutual fund of the faculty member's choice.

Defined contribution plans generally have a mandatory participation provision and a mandatory minimum employee contribution. There are usually opportunities to contribute beyond the mandatory employee contribution, and most financial experts advise clients to take advantage of any *voluntary opportunities* to contribute beyond the mandated contribution. Such opportunities have the obvious advantage of deferring more income and allowing such deferrals to grow tax-free over time.

In theory, and referring back to the *time value of money*, these *regular contributions* to a *diversified investment account* will grow to a sizeable amount of money that will adequately fund a faculty member's retirement. One of the keys to success with this type of plan is to begin saving early and often. One advantage of such a defined contribution plan is that the faculty member can choose how the funds are invested, a choice that will eventually affect the total retirement funds available upon retirement. Also, the faculty member can choose how much to draw out of the account in any given retirement year, but such decisions have tax consequences; that is, withdraw too little and tax penalties are incurred, while withdrawing too much results in higher taxes as the faculty member's income moves up into higher tax brackets. A disadvantage to the plan becomes evident when the faculty member starts saving too late, or makes poor investment choices, thereby diminishing the amount of funds available upon retirement.

On a final note about retirement plans, the faculty member might come across the term "*vested*." According to the US

Department of Labor, individuals are "vested" after they have a right to funds that have been invested on their behalf or when they are fully eligible for the retirement plan benefits. "Vesting" can be immediate or occur in increments toward "full vesting" over a period of time [10].

Personal Investment Management

In addition to annual income, another component of "Me, Inc." is the smart management of investments and other income both now and into the future. As noted above, it is likely the annual salary and commensurate benefits attached to the faculty member's position that will contribute to building an investment portfolio. Certainly other household income such as a spouse's potential salary, inheritance, outside consulting, and other income may also contribute to a household net worth.

Building savings and investments is a function of one's stage in life. It is not uncommon for individuals early in their career to begin with a negative net worth (more liabilities than assets) but then watch their net worth change to the positive as their career progresses, annual income grows, loans get paid off, homes are purchased and savings plans mature.

Financial advisors often suggest thinking of savings in at least two "buckets," with one bucket identified for the short-term. The common rule of thumb for this bucket is 3–6 months of readily accessible cash that can adequately cover monthly living expenses in the case of job loss, a health or other life event or other unplanned emergency. The general investment tools recommended for such savings are generally low-risk and can be easily redeemable certificates of deposit, money market and other cash-type savings accounts.

The second bucket of savings is for the long term (also known as "retirement" in this instance). Because these types of savings and investments are intended to extend over decades, they are generally in accounts less accessible, generally carry financial penalties if accessed prematurely, and often carry more risk, to achieve maximal growth. As noted earlier, 401(k), 403(b) and 457(b) plans are the most common deferred compensation tools used to save for the long-term. These plans have the advantage of setting aside pre-tax income into the account and also the advantage of tax-deferred growth while the funds are in the account.

Two other common methods to shelter income and save for the long term are the Individual Retirement Account (IRA) and the Roth IRA. The former allows for sheltering annual income on a pre- and after-tax basis and deferring taxes until withdrawals occur while the latter Roth IRA allows for after-tax sheltering of funds that will grow in a tax deferred manner but also allows for tax-free withdrawals. When using such investment tactics, investors need to remain mindful of Internal Revenue Service definitions and limits on eligible contributions for all types of tax deferred retirement savings.

The level of *financial risk* and the degree of *financial diversity* that an investment portfolio contains are key contributors to how fast and how much the retirement accounts will grow. Low-risk investments such as passbook savings, money market accounts and savings, and other types of bonds can be secure, but the trade-off for that security is lower returns and slower growth over the long term. Adding more risk and diversity to the investment portfolio will create higher returns, but also be less secure, especially in the short-term. Higher risk often means higher volatility in the investment account so it is always important for investors to understand their level of risk tolerance, the length of time the funds will be invested and the ultimate goal of the investment account.

Such analysis requires time and expertise, and in the absence of both, as noted earlier, there are a variety of financial experts who can assist with such thinking and analysis.

Personal Risk Management

When running the business of "Me, Inc." the faculty member, as would any good Chief Executive Officer, must consider how to manage the risk of the enterprise—in this instance, personal risk. The Oxford English Dictionary defines *risk* as "the possibility that something unpleasant or unwelcome will happen" [11]. Many of the chapters of this book deal with the concept of managing and developing one's professional life. This chapter involves financial concepts related to one's personal life and protecting "Me, Inc.'s" personal wealth and loved ones from the possibility of something unpleasant or unwelcome.

Risk is a concept that has been around for generations and, as a result, the solutions available to manage risk have been around almost as long. Like any good strategy, risk management is not one "thing" but, rather, a set of programs designed to complement each other. As the paragraphs below illustrate, personal risk management generally involves a combination of insurance (professional liability, life, home, auto, umbrellas, etc.) and well-drafted legal documents that anticipate one's incapacity or death. Each one of these is a necessary tool to a well-developed risk management strategy.

Insurance as a Risk Management Strategy

Insuring risk is a time-tested method of managing the potential of personal calamity. Some types of insurance are mandated by law or by the ordinary course of business; other, less common types, are a matter of personal preference or (as will be shown below) are simply good practice. While the list of coverages one should consider may seem overwhelming, and the cost imposing, the risk of doing nothing and the potential downside of an insurable event are far more problematic.

Professional Liability Insurance

Faculty physicians and other faculty clinical providers are at risk for their own professional conduct. In a litigious society, clinical providers are held to very high standards and, rightly or wrongly, blamed for bad things that happen to their patients. While the psychological damage that results from being sued for malpractice can be great, the financial loss can be devastating. In order to protect patients, as well as to protect clinical providers, most states require practicing clinicians to carry certain minimum amounts of *professional liability coverage*. For example, in order to maintain a license to practice medicine in the State of Wisconsin, a doctor must carry liability insurance with coverage limits of $1 million per occurrence and $3 million in the aggregate (annually) [12]. In addition, he or she must also participate in the so-called "Patients Compensation Fund" maintained by the State of Wisconsin to pay for damages in excess of the above-described coverage limits [12].

As one might imagine, the cost of this type of insurance can be high, and in some states with active plaintiff's bars, difficult to obtain. In most instances this insurance will be mandated and procured by the faculty clinician's employer. Depending upon the faculty compensation plan in place, the cost of this insurance may be considered general overhead, factored into the physician's overhead computation when calculating incentives, or less frequently, the cost can simply be deducted from his or her salary.

Health and Long-Term Disability Coverage

Other critical components of a personal insurance strategy are *health and disability insurance*. With recent changes to federal law, specifically those occasioned by the Patient Protection and Affordable Care Act of 2010 (PPACA), each person over the age of 26 is legally required to maintain health insurance, and insurers are required to provide coverage regardless of pre-existing conditions (At the time of this writing, there are a number of legal challenges to the so-called "individual mandate" found in the PPACA). Luckily and as noted earlier, for most faculty in academic medical center settings, health insurance is an employment benefit provided by employers. The cost of all, or some, of this insurance is likely to be paid for by the academic institution and, likely, the remainder by the faculty member through payroll deductions. It is noteworthy that the high cost of health insurance and the changes required by the PPACA have resulted in creative arrangements that will allow an insured to hold down his or her individual cost. For example, many insurers now offer "high deductible" plans, which place the risk of the first $1500–$5000 of health care costs on the insured. In many cases these deductibles can be paid for with pre-tax dollars through health savings accounts (referred to as "HSAs" and discussed earlier), reducing further the cost of health insurance and, as noted earlier, lowering taxable income.

Closely related to health insurance is *disability insurance*. While health insurance pays medical costs, it does not replace the income lost due to one's inability to work because of a medical condition. Should one become ill or injured and, as a result, not able to work for long periods of time, personal wealth can be quickly depleted. Disability insurance can help manage this risk by paying the disabled person a portion of his or her income in the event of a disability. As noted earlier, this insurance will usually be offered as part of an employment package and, if not, is available from a variety of private insurers. That said, there are pros and cons to carrying disability insurance.

As noted above, disability coverage replaces income lost due to the inability to work, thus protecting savings, investments and other assets, such as home equity. Moreover, insurance payments from private insurers should not affect the ability to obtain government disability benefits, such as those paid by Social Security. In addition, if disability insurance premiums are paid with after-tax dollars, disability benefits should not be taxable. That said, disability insurance premiums are not inexpensive. The average cost of group coverage is approximately $250 per month and can be higher if purchased on an individual basis [13]. In addition, should premiums be paid with pre-tax dollars or by an employer, some or all of the benefit payments will be taxable. In addition, most will have to wait up to 4 months in order to start receiving benefits, during which time living expenses will need to be covered by personal savings should the faculty member's employer fail to continue salary during that waiting period (please note that for faculty physicians, many employment agreements provide for salary continuation during the waiting period prior to a finding of permanent disability). Finally, disability insurance does not cover 100 % of lost income (and contains a "hard cap" on total payments) and is not a permanent solution as very few policies provide benefits beyond normal retirement age [14].

Life Insurance

In general, *life insurance* is designed to replace lost income, and take care of one's dependents and loved ones, in the event of the death of the insured. The amount of insurance and the type of insurance one may decide to carry, if carried at all, often is a matter of debate.

In general, there are two types of life insurance: *term* and *whole (or universal) life. Term* insurance is considered a "pure" type of insurance; the faculty member's life is insured for a large sum of money and all premiums paid are retained by the insurance company and used to cover the cost of insurance, and the payout, should one occur. Generally, as soon as life insurance payments for premiums cease, term life insurance coverage simultaneously terminates. Because it builds no cash value, term insurance is usually less expensive than *whole life* insurance, a product offered by many insurance and financial services companies containing both a "pure" insurance component and an "investment" component.

A whole life insurance policy increases in value over time as a result of the investment component and can be surrendered for its cash value or the cash value can be used to continue to pay the whole life insurance premiums at some point in the future.

Because of the investment component, whole life insurance is substantially more expensive than term coverage. The debate between term and whole life coverage is whether or not whole life is worth the extra cost. Many financial experts believe that one should buy term insurance and simply invest the difference between the cost of term and whole life. Conversely, other experts will tout the investment performance—sometimes guaranteed—of their whole life insurance product and the current tax-deferred growth it offers. The question for most is whether or not the insured believes that the insurance company can invest his or her money better, and cheaper, than can he or she.

In addition to the type of insurance to be purchased, the amount of insurance coverage also has to be considered. This question is not as easy as it might sound. There are a substantial number of factors that go into this determination, such as age, the amount of personal wealth owned by the insured and its liquidity, the number and age of dependents and the debts left upon death. Be careful about relying on "rules of thumb" such as buying six-to-eight time's annual income as one may find him or herself over, or under, insured. The academic faculty member is well counseled to consider his or her personal circumstances and needs before buying insurance and, only then, buying accordingly.

Home, Auto and Umbrella Insurance

If one owns a home, and carries a mortgage on that home, the mortgage lender will require that the *home be insured*. Even if the home is owned free and clear of mortgages, it is wise practice to carry insurance on the home and its contents. A *standard homeowner's policy* will cover the home and personal effects, as well as the homeowner's liability for injuries or property damage caused to others by the homeowner, his or her family members or pets. Most policies also provide additional dollars to cover living expenses in case the home cannot be lived in while it is being repaired. In this regard, it is important to understand what a policy covers and what it does not cover. Most policies are designed to cover all "*perils*" other than those specifically excluded in the policy. Before one purchases homeowner's insurance, he or she should read the policy, or have it explained. In most cases, homeowner's policies do not cover events such as earthquakes or floods, risks which must be separately insured. In addition to the above, it is important to understand coverage limits. Most insurance experts advise that the cost to rebuild the home should be insured, not its market value. This is especially important during times where market values have dropped dramatically, such as since 2008.

Nowadays, most states require that an automobile driver carry insurance. To be clear, *automobile insurance* is not insurance on the car; it is insurance on the driver. There are, generally, three types of automotive insurance: *personal liability and personal damage, comprehensive and collision. Personal liability* and *personal damage coverage* (PLPD) generally only cover personal liability and personal damage for which the driver is responsible. It will not, however, cover vehicle repairs or replacement of the vehicle. This type of coverage is, generally, the cheapest form of auto insurance. *Comprehensive and collision insurance*, on the other hand, is considered "full" coverage and will cover the driver as well as the other people and property involved in an incident. For example, collision insurance covers the cost of repairs or replacement for the vehicle and property caused by a collision. Comprehensive covers losses from situations other than collisions. These types of insurance are, often, more wise to carry than simple PLPD coverage, but of course, are more expensive. As with home-owner's coverage, it is important to understand what is, and is not, covered. For example, the cost of towing, a rental car and medical care arising out of an auto accident generally are not covered and must be separately insured.

Closely related to home and auto coverage, and worth consider-ing should personal wealth or earnings be significant, is "*umbrella*" *coverage. Umbrella* coverage will protect the insured from major claims and lawsuits by providing additional liability coverage above the limits of homeowners and auto policies. For example, if a faculty member or family member is at fault in an auto accident and the other party is badly injured and incurs damages exceeding limits of the automotive policy, the faculty member's personal assets could be at risk for such excess loss unless umbrella cover-age is carried. In this instance, if there were a loss incurred above the limits of the insured's automotive policy's bodily injury cover-age, an umbrella policy would cover the excess loss. Umbrella policies are generally carried with coverage limits of no less than $1,000,000 and are relatively affordable.

Other Risk Management Tools

In addition to insurance coverage, there are several other effective, and relatively simple, ways to manage personal risk: developing *powers of attorney* (such as *financial* and *health care powers of attorney*) and creating a *will*. Each of these legal instruments will provide those around the faculty member with instructions as to what to do if he or she is too ill to direct his or her own affairs and, further, give them certainty relative to the faculty member's affairs and estate following his or her death.

Health care powers of attorney are becoming increasingly common and come in several forms. This instrument, usually prepared by an attorney, will direct one or more persons (who will act as the faculty member's agent(s)) to make decisions on behalf of a person regarding his or her medical care in the event they are no longer able to make or communicate those decisions. The benefits of a well designed document are many, and the downsides of drafting and maintaining such an instrument are few (if any).

Most health care powers of attorney give the faculty member's agent the authority to make decisions and communicate with doctors, hospitals, nursing homes or health care facilities and any other health care personnel. A standard health care power of attorney gives the agent the authority to, among other things, consent to the administration of pain relieving drugs and to any treatment the agent believes is in the best interests of the person under medical care and consistent with such person's wishes, withdraw or consent to life-sustaining treatment in the event that the person under care is in a terminal condition, request copies of and review health care records, disclose those records and information to others and select and employ health care providers.

The form of a power of attorney can be as simple or as detailed as one wishes. As should be evident from the discussion above, the document will provide loved ones with a degree of certainty as to what to do in the event a person cannot direct his or her own care. Moreover, a well-drafted power of attorney can help ease some of the emotional burden of an already strained situation and, further, may help ameliorate costly bickering among family members and unnecessary legal fees occasioned by health care providers seeking "cover" for their decisions relative to the care of someone who is unable to direct that care. A financial power of attorney functions in much the same way as does a health care power of attorney. Rather than allowing the agent to direct medical care and treatment decisions, the financial power of attorney allows one's agent to direct and take care of financial matters.

A final, necessary, component of a personal risk mitigation strategy is the preparation of a *will*. The primary purpose of a will is to direct the distribution of one's assets (often referred to as an "*estate*") in the event of death. Should a person die without a will—known as dying "*intestate*"—the distribution of most, if not all, of the deceased's assets will be guided by state law, which may be contrary to a person's actual wishes (were he or she to be alive). By creating a will, the CEO of "Me, Inc.," again, creates a level of certainty for those whom he or she leaves behind. A will directs the distribution of a person's estate and ensures that those who are to receive his or her assets, or the income or distributions from those assets, receive them. In addition, if properly prepared in conjunction with a thoughtful estate plan, a will can mitigate the effect of, what can be, devastating estate taxes, thereby preserving the value of the assets passed along to a spouse, children and others. Dying without a will, or dying with a poorly constructed will, can result in assets being distributed contrary to one's wishes, cost the estate vast sums of money (lost to state and federal taxes) or devolve into family fights over assets; clearly not a legacy one would wish to leave.

Most will agree that personal risk management is not pleasant and it is not inexpensive. However, when done thoughtfully and carefully it can mitigate the cost and loss resulting from an unwanted or unpleasant event. Moreover, smart risk management can provide one's family, friends and loved ones with peace of mind should the unfortunate happen.

Conclusion

"Me, Inc." is really a complex business comprised of annual income management, investment management and risk management. Each of these areas, with their own complexities, requires careful thought and consideration, all with the goal of ensuring financial security and supporting a personally and professionally robust and satisfying life.

Smartly managing personal income by knowing and understanding the full range of benefits offered by the academic employer is a key component toward this goal. Faculty need to take advantage of every opportunity the employer offers to contribute to his or her financial well-being, either through enrolling in benefits, deferring salaried income and joining various insurance plans.

Moving beyond the base salary, faculty need to think about saving and investing for both the short and long term. Understanding different investment tools, how to maximize savings through tax-deferred investments combined with the right mixture of risk and diversity, is a must.

Finally, recognizing first that there are risks in life and then understanding the different ways to manage and plan for these risks is a critical feature of managing personal finances. Protecting members of the academic household, ensuring against catastrophic events and developing an end-of-life plan are part of risk management and the last essential component of a "Me, Inc."

The faculty member who remembers some general rules of thumb, seeks advice when necessary, thinks in both the short and long term and has a risk management plan in place for the unforeseen, unknown or unexpected event will do well.

Words to the Wise
- Review wills, durable powers of attorney and beneficiary information in such documents as insurance policies regularly.
- Check investment portfolios regularly, but not too often. After establishing and asset allocation strategy, checking portfolios no often than quarterly or semi-annually is generally recommended, but no less than annually. This minimizes the risk of overreacting to transient news and events.
- The cost of hiring an attorney to design a simple will and establish powers of attorney varies by city and region but will likely cost between $1000 and $2000.
- "Virtual banks" (no bricks and mortar) can be an effective way to maximize interest earnings on savings accounts, but these banks can be more restrictive with withdrawals and the frequency of the same.
- Credit Unions are often more consumer friendly and can offer affordable house and auto loans and can also offer marginally better interest rates on savings accounts and certificates of deposit.

(continued)

(continued)

• Know your comfort level with risk. The tolerance for risk can change with the stages of life where more risk can be tolerated early in a career and less risk is recommended for later in a career and retirement.

Ask Your Mentor or Colleagues
• What happens if I don't contribute to a retirement plan?
• Who should I consult when performing some estate planning?
• What value does an accountant or financial advisor add to my financial planning? Do I need either?
• Do I really need all of these insurances described in the chapter?

References

1. David J. Peterson, "Taking Care of Me, Inc.," AAP Grapevine 12, no.1 (Winter 1999): 11.
2. National Vital Statistics Reports, Vol. 59, No. 9 September 28, 2011; available at http://www.cdc.gov/nchs/data/nvsr/nvsr59/nvsr59_09.pdf.
3. MarketWatch: The Big Chill – A Look at Boomers' Top 10 Desired Retirement Activities; available at http://www.marketwatch.com/story/story/print?guid=AEB55911-079E-4B68-8FEF-5A465EE3A0E7.
4. O. Maurice Joy, Introduction to Financial Management (Homewood, Ill.: Richard D. Irwin, Inc., 1980), 47–64.
5. Rule of 72 Definition; available at http://www.investopedia.com/terms/r/ruleof72.asp#axzzldQETdS7W.
6. CNN Money: Good debt vs. bad debt; available at http://money.cnn.com/magazines/moneymag/money101/lesson9/indexz.htm.
7. Investopedia: Pay Yourself first; available at http://www.investopedia.com/terms/p/payourselffirst.asp#axzzldQETdS7W.
8. CNN Money: Top things to know; available at http://money.cnn.com/magazines/moneymag/money101/lesson15/index.htm.

9. US Securities and Exchange Commission, Beginners Guide to Asset allocation, Diversification and Rebalancing; available at http://www.sec.gov/investor/pubs/assetallocation.htm.
10. US Department of Labor, Employee Benefits Security Administration, What You Should Know About Your Retirement; available at http://www.dol.gov.ebsa/publications/wyskzpr.html.
11. Oxford English Dictionary (2nd Edition).
12. Wis. Stat. Chap. 655.
13. JHA US Group Disability Market Survey; available at http://www.genre.com/sharedfile/pdf/GDMYS200608-en.pdf.
14. Smart Money, Do You need Disability Insurance; available at http://www.smartmoney.com/plan/insurance/do-you-need-disability-insurance-17318/.

How to Create Your Package for Promotion

7

Judith P. Cain and David K. Stevenson

From the perspective of the candidate, the pathways leading to the promotion review—as well as the review itself—are often seen as mysterious and confusing. This observation was confirmed in a 2008 study conducted by the Collaborative on Academic Careers in Higher Education (COACHE) [1] in which pre-tenure faculty at medical schools and health professions gave low ratings to the level of clarity surrounding tenure processes, criteria, standards, and the body of evidence needed for promotion.

Some of this mystery and confusion is complicated by the subjective, evaluative aspect of promotion standards. In that respect, there are no easy answers to such questions as the following: How many peer-reviewed articles do I need? When, what, and where should I publish? What types of grants and how much funding should I have? How many students should I be teaching and mentoring? What ratings do I have to have on my teaching and clinical evaluations? Also, academic careers tend to be individualized in terms of breadth, depth, and focus, resulting in multiple pathways

J.P. Cain (✉)
Department of Medicine, Stanford University,
1265 Welch Road, Stanford, CA, USA
e-mail: jpcain@stanford.edu

© Springer International Publishing Switzerland 2016
L.W. Roberts (ed.), *The Associate Professor Guidebook*,
DOI 10.1007/978-3-319-28001-1_7

to success. Thus, it is difficult, if not impossible, to draw a specific road map that can be universally applied to all faculty that will predict or guarantee a successful promotion outcome.

The application of promotion criteria is usually centered on expectations for excellence in a particular faculty line. For example, in the tenure line, a greater proportional weight may be given to scholarship than in a more clinically-oriented line where there may be a balance between clinical care, teaching, and scholarly activities; in some lines, senior-authored, peer-reviewed publications are the *coin of the realm*, while in others there may be more flexibility in considering collaborative work, case reports, invited chapters, textbooks, or conference proceedings. Chapter 7 provides guidance in understanding criteria for *traditional*, *research*, *clinical educator*, and *teaching* tracks. In addition to evaluating achievements against the criteria for a specific line, those reviewing the promotion package will be assessing the relative placement within a field or subfield nationally; Chap. 8 will be helpful in mapping out a plan to build a national reputation.

Given that there is no single prescribed, quantifiable path to promotion, perceptions regarding criteria and standards can be influenced by a variety of experiences, both personal and professional. As a result, different things may be said by different people about what is needed to advance in rank. While it will be important to gather perspectives from a variety of individuals in the years leading up to the promotion review, under most circumstances—and since the review will be initiated at the departmental level—the department chair is in the best position to provide guidance and counsel, to confirm current standards, and to interpret how the criteria will be applied in considering a particular case for promotion.

Institutional Responsibility

Institutions share the common goal of creating a culture and building an environment in which their faculty can develop, flourish, and succeed. In response to the COACHE study, and as part of a continuing commitment to enhance professional development opportunities for early-career faculty, many institutions have made it a priority to promote accessibility, clarity, and transparency in promotion reviews. Toward that end, efforts have included making policy documents (such as faculty handbooks) widely and easily available; offering university-, school-, or department-sponsored workshops on promotion criteria and processes; developing flexible workplace arrangements that may include extension of the promotion clock; initiating annual pre-promotion discussions between the department chair (or designate) and the early-career faculty member in order to regularly assess the candidate's progress toward promotion; providing training sessions for departmental, school, and university review committees; and actively protecting and preserving the integrity of the evaluation process by carefully following standardized procedures.

Of course, institutional responsibility is also carried out on a more direct and personal level. Through its decision to hire a new faculty member, the department has expressed its confidence not only in the individual's past and present achievements but also in his or her promise for the future. Because of this investment in the faculty member's success, the department chair, senior colleagues, and mentors will be partners in his or her professional development, providing support and honest assessment of career development and progress as the person moves through the early years of appointment.

Faculty Responsibility

While institutions have certain obligations, it is important for faculty to understand that they must be active in preparing for promotion and take responsibility for their career trajectory. As the primary stakeholder in the process, faculty should actively seek out information that will assist in the promotion process. The investment of time and effort in learning as much as possible about what is expected can pay dividends later. The confidence that comes with understanding the promotion process will enable faculty to put forth a promotion package that makes a compelling case for advancement.

Building a Strong Foundation of Knowledge

It is always a good idea to establish a baseline of information early. Candidates should reread their offer letter for details about faculty line, responsibilities, appointment term, and criteria for reappointment or promotion. They should study their institution's faculty handbook (usually readily available online), which will be an invaluable resource in providing information about the fundamentals of criteria, policies, and procedures. School or departmental websites may also provide useful information, especially with respect to any supplemental practices at those levels. A variety of other information may also be posted on these websites, such as the components of the promotion package (including the candidate's contributions), sample letters used in soliciting evaluations from referees and trainees, sample teaching and clinical evaluation forms, and timelines. If anything is unclear, especially regarding promotion criteria, the candidate should seek out answers from departmental leadership sooner rather than later.

Although the actual promotion review may be years in the future, it is important that the candidate systematically records and tracks relevant achievements as they occur. Faculty at many institutions have access to vendor or in-house web databases for the creation of e-portfolios. This is an efficient and productive way to store and update the curriculum vitae, annual activity reports, and other information on scholarly, teaching, and clinical activities that will be needed for the midterm and promotion reviews. Understanding the scope of and required formats for these materials will allow the candidate to collect and organize information cumulatively rather than at the last minute.

As mentioned previously, many institutions offer orientations or regular workshops for faculty focusing on such topics as promotion criteria, timing, and dossier preparation. Candidates for promotion should make every effort to participate in such sessions; if they are unable to attend, they should ask for copies of the slides or handouts from the meeting and follow up with questions, if necessary. They should also be alert to other workshops that may be held on such topics as time management, work–life balance, negotiating skills, and networking within and beyond the boundaries of their institution, all of which are aimed at enhancing professional development and success as a member of the academic community.

Annual meetings with the department chair or designate will provide a regular opportunity to discuss and measure progress against criteria for promotion. If such annual meetings are not common practice in their department, faculty members should initiate them. This is particularly important in the early years of the appointment since such sessions will provide ample time to address any issues and, if necessary, make course corrections well in advance of the promotion review. Mentors can also provide guidance and counsel and be good sounding boards as the candidate moves through the first, second, and third years of appointment.

The Midterm Review and Beyond

Typically, candidates will have a formal review of their performance near the midpoint of the appointment. For assistant professors who are on a 7-year appointment track, this review will be conducted in either the third or fourth year of appointment. At many institutions, the midterm evaluation is not as extensive as the promotion review but shares some of the same elements and thus can serve as a useful preview. Feedback from the review should be used to address any concerns and to build momentum that will carry the candidate through promotion review 3 or 4 years hence.

After the midterm review, efforts should be stepped up to gather perspectives that will be of value and benefit as the promotion review draws closer. Those who have invested in the candidate's success, including the department chair or division leader, senior colleagues, and mentors, will all be in a position to provide targeted, strategic counseling and feedback. Departmental or school administrative staff will be able to provide technical advice about the process. Colleagues within or outside the department who have recently been promoted may be willing to share their experiences. Senior faculty who have completed terms of service on school or university review committees may be able to provide insight into what distinguishes a superb promotion dossier from a weak one. It is important to note that under most circumstances, it is considered inappropriate to approach faculty currently serving in such a role and inquire about the disposition of a particular dossier (see Table 7.1).

Table 7.1 Sample pathway to the promotion review

Year 1	Re-read offer letter; study faculty handbook; review relevant websites, create an electronic portfolio to record and track achievements systematically
Year 2	Attend promotion workshops; meet frequently with mentor(s); meet with department chair annually to discuss progress toward promotion
Year 3	Understand policies regarding promotion clock extensions; prepare materials for midterm review
Year 4	Midterm review
Year 5	Incorporate and act on feedback from midterm review
Year 6	Continue regular meetings with mentor(s) and annual meetings with department chair; initiate conversations with those recently promoted; seek strategic advice from senior colleagues
Year 7	Begin preparation of promotion package; circulate CV and candidate's statement for feedback; submit promotion package

Timing of the Promotion Review

In order to prepare for the promotion review, candidates need to be familiar with issues surrounding timing. The length of the appointment term—and therefore the timing of the promotion review—may depend on which faculty line the candidate is in. For example, in the School of Medicine at Stanford University, early-career faculty who are in the University Tenure Line (with a primary emphasis on research and teaching) typically have an initial appointment of 4 years followed by reappointment for 3 years; the tenure review is then initiated at the beginning of the seventh year in rank. Faculty in the Medical Center Line (where there is an expectation for excellence in the overall mix of clinical care, research, and teaching) are on a 10-year appointment clock, with an initial appointment of 4 years followed by a 6-year reappointment; the promotion review starts at the beginning of the tenth year.

At many institutions, there is often flexibility around extending the appointment end date for faculty who become new parents. Early on, faculty members should learn about this or any other circumstances that might result in favorable consideration of such an extension. On the other end of the spectrum, there may be flexibility regarding consideration for early promotion. Coming up early for promotion or extending the timing of the decision both require advance planning and close consultation with the department chair.

Typically, the promotion review will be launched up to 1 year in advance of the candidate's appointment end date. Timelines will vary institution by institution but are influenced by a common set of rate-limiting requirements, including the often lengthy process of soliciting and receiving letters from referees, students, and trainees; gathering, presenting, and evaluating evidence regarding scholarship, teaching, and clinical activities; and multiple levels of evaluation by departmental, school, and university review committees. All of this can and does take time. A sample timeline of the promotion process is included in the Appendix.

One of the topics at the midterm review should be the timing of the promotion review. Candidates will need to know not only the date when their department will formally launch the review but also the approximate deadline for submission of materials, which will allow them to plan accordingly. For example, if candidates are on a 7-year promotion clock, their review could be initiated as early as the *beginning* of the seventh year of appointment. Given the demands on their time, they should normally allow between 3 and 6 months to assemble the promotion package. They may need less, but it is better to provide the luxury of a *cushion*.

Candidates for promotion have the responsibility for designing and pursuing a schedule of research that results in publication in advance of the promotion review. Generally, by the time materials have been submitted, the candidate's dossier should predominantly reflect a record of actual accomplishment (which confirms status in the field) rather than work that has been submitted or accepted but not yet published (which may speak more to promise). Similarly, the faculty member's career should be managed so that teaching and clinical care records are robust and ready to be evaluated by the time that the promotion package is submitted.

Review committee members will expect expert referees to assess the candidate's impact and influence as a scholar through the lens of work that has been subjected to broad, formal scrutiny and cited by leaders in the field. Although unpublished work cannot be evaluated in the same way, it is important to document works in progress in the curriculum vitae and personal statement as this will be valuable in confirming momentum and upward trajectory.

Along with understanding the timing of the review, it is also important to be on time in submitting promotion materials. Candidate-driven delays can raise issues of professionalism at a highly inopportune time. If there are compelling reasons why a candidate is unable to meet any deadlines for submission of the dossier, the department chair should be informed immediately.

The Components of the Promotion Package

From evaluations by referees and students to departmental commentary and analysis of a candidate's contributions, there are many interconnected components of the promotion review. Its centerpiece, however, is the candidate's contribution, which provides an opportunity to both showcase accomplishments and to illuminate future plans. Sometimes called a *dossier* or *portfolio*, such contributions will typically include:

Curriculum Vitae

Chapter 5 of this book focuses on how to prepare the best possible curriculum vitae when joining a faculty. Building on that strong foundation, here are some things that candidates should consider when preparing a CV for the promotion review:

– Build the CV systematically and over time, using online tools to collect and track accomplishments and contributions.
– If the institution requires a standardized format, use it.
– Review sample CVs on departmental or school websites or ask recently promoted colleagues if they would be willing to share their CV.
– Distinguish between peer-reviewed and non-peer-reviewed publications and between invited presentations (even those declined) and *call for papers*. Those who will be reviewing the promotion package will be expecting this distinction, and not making it can create confusion or give the impression that the candidate is mischaracterizing his or her contributions.

- Authorship practices in many disciplines follow a traditional pattern in which the first author listed is the primary author and the last author listed is the senior author associated with the work. If practices differ in a discipline, this should be explained in a footnote or in the candidate's statement.
- Note which publications are in press and which have been submitted and to whom.
- For teaching contributions, use a broad definition that includes the classroom, laboratory or clinical setting, advising, mentoring, program building, and curricular innovation.
- In addition to clinical contributions that are reflected through scholarly and teaching activities, such things as medical consultancies, hospital appointments, and patents should be highlighted.
- There is a fine line between being comprehensive and padding the CV; candidates should learn the difference by concentrating on substantive contributions and, if uncertain, ask the department chair, mentor, or colleagues for advice.
- If responsibility for keeping the CV up to date has been delegated to administrative staff, candidates should remember that they are ultimately responsible for its content. The document should be read thoroughly and proofread by at least one other person.

With the increasing prevalence of *team science*, it can be challenging for committee reviewers to determine the nature of individual substantive contributions to multi-author works when reviewing a CV. Under such circumstances, candidates might want to consider briefly annotating selected bibliographic entries to highlight individual contributions to collaborative efforts.

A version of authorship requirements of the *Journal of the American Medical Association* [2], which includes the following categories, can be used as a model: (1) conception and design, acquisition of data and analysis and interpretation of data; (2) drafting of the manuscript and critical revision of the manuscript for important intellectual content; and (3) statistical analysis, obtaining funding, administrative, technical or material support, and supervision.

Candidates should anticipate that file reviewers will notice if there are unusual gaps in their CV and provide context for this in their candidate's statement. For example, a shift in research direction may have influenced productivity, the rate of publications flowing out of clinical trials may have been slowed due to lengthy periods of design and implementation, or sanctioned periods of protected time for research may have resulted in a reduced number of teaching opportunities. In providing this information, the tone should be explanatory and not defensive.

Candidate's Statement

Sometimes called the *personal* or *self* statement, this document serves as the candidate's voice in the promotion review and as a rich resource to those evaluating the case for promotion. In this narrative report, candidates will have an opportunity to discuss their accomplishments to date, the intersections of their scholarly, teaching, and clinical care contributions, and their plans for the future. Inclusion of a candidate's statement in the promotion package is sometimes optional but is almost always a good investment of time and effort. More often than not, institutions will have a required format, as well as page limitations. Knowing this well in advance will provide candidates with a framework in which to craft and effectively present their case for promotion.

There will be multiple audiences for the candidate's statement. Some readers, including departmental colleagues and external referees, will have expertise in and an understanding of the evolution of the candidate's discipline. Others, including members of school and university review committees, the dean, and the provost, may have homes in disciplines further removed from or entirely outside of academic medicine (such as physics, economics, or history). Because of this, candidates should take care to describe their accomplishments in lay terms that will be understandable and accessible to those outside their field.

With the caveat that the faculty member's department will be the primary source for information regarding the content and format of the candidate's statement, the following general guidelines may prove useful:

- While it is often appropriate to include contextual information regarding earlier contributions, it is usually important to concentrate on achievements made during the current term of appointment. For example, if the candidate is being reviewed at the beginning of the seventh year of appointment, accomplishments realized over the last 5 or 6 years may prove most relevant for purposes of evaluating satisfaction of criteria for promotion.

- In order to provide evaluators with a sense of career trajectory, it is important to include a discussion of near-term (e.g., works in progress), longer-range plans and goals for future work.
- Commentary should be included for each area on which the candidate will be evaluated, and the statement should be organized to align with the relative weight given to promotion criteria. For example, if the candidate will be evaluated primarily on clinical care activities (and, presumably, the highest proportion of time is dedicated to that area), the candidate's statement should begin with that and then, in descending order of weight and contribution, address other areas of contribution.
- The section on scholarly activities might include a general description of the overall investigative program, major contributions and accomplishments with particular emphasis on recent achievements, major publications and scientific discoveries and how they have impacted knowledge or further research in the field and/or patient care (including those that rank highly on citation indices), major grants and awards, and future goals, including ongoing research projects, publications planned for submission, and grant applications planned or in review.
- As mentioned previously, if authorship practices in the faculty member's discipline vary from the norm, this should be explained in the candidate's statement.
- The section on teaching might include commentary on clinical *bedside* teaching (e.g., medical students, residents, fellows, ancillary staff, and visiting or community physicians); didactic instruction, including informal lectures in the clinical setting, formal classroom lectures, and continuing education; career mentoring and advising contributions; research mentoring and director supervision (undergraduate students, graduate students, postdoctoral fellows, medical students, residents, clinical fellows); prestigious positions obtained by former

trainees; program or curriculum development; teaching awards; and future goals and plans.

– Commentary on clinical care activities could include discussion of the candidate's area of expertise and inpatient/outpatient/ procedural contributions, percentages of time spent in clinic or the operating room, interaction with or consultation to other services, outreach contributions, development and/or imple- mentation of new clinical trials or protocols and their real or potential impact, grand rounds, clinical care awards received, and future goals and plans.

– Some institutions protect early-career faculty from administra- tive commitments but, if relevant and applicable to promotion criteria, a description of service roles, responsibilities, and accomplishments should be included.

– In cases where promotion criteria include regional or national recognition, service positions (e.g., editorial or grant reviewer), major invited presentations or visiting professorships, confer- ences and symposia organized, and elected leadership positions and/or honors and awards from professional societies should be highlighted.

Sample Publications

Many institutions require or encourage submission of work, usu- ally in the form of publications, as part of the promotion package. In some cases, such samples are shared locally, that is, with depart- mental faculty and/or departmental school and university evalua- tion committees. In other cases, a candidate's publications will also be sent to external referees. Since the number of publications to be submitted is usually limited, it is important that they be selected with thoughtfulness and care.

Normally, sample publications will be those that have appeared in print. Occasionally, however, there may be compelling reasons to include submitted or accepted publications that are unpub- lished at the time of the promotion review. Candidates are encour- aged to seek guidance from the department chair, mentor, or senior colleagues in this matter.

Educator Portfolio

An *educator* or *teaching* portfolio is sometimes a required component of the promotion package. As with the curriculum vitae and candidate's statement, there may be a prescribed format, which should be followed closely.

Referees

Candidates for promotion are often asked to provide the names of leaders in the field who would be in a position to evaluate their work. The composition of the referee set varies by institution but may include a combination of mentors or collaborators of the candidate as well as those who are at *arm's length* and can provide independent perspectives. Colleagues within the candidate's institution may also be asked to provide a letter of evaluation.

For many reasons, including opportunities for advancement in their career, it is important for faculty members to be active and visible members of their discipline through participating in conferences and symposia, making presentations to national audiences, and serving on review panels and editorial boards. Likewise, it is crucial to establish, build, and sustain strong relationships with departmental colleagues and, given the evolving interdisciplinary nature of many fields, to make connections across other departments. Through such networking activities, the candidate will be well positioned to suggest the names of referees who are familiar with his or her work and will be able to provide a substantive and meaningful evaluation.

Post-submission of the Promotion Package

After materials have been submitted, departmental staff will contact the candidate if questions arise. If significant events—such as grants, publication acceptances, or awards—occur *after* the promotion package has been submitted, candidates should check with their department chair to see if there is a way for this information to become part of the record under review.

In the interest of transparency and clarity, the department chair should be able to provide the candidate with an approximate time-line for the final decision. Depending on an institution's policies, this could be either weeks or months, although the candidate may be informed at intervals as the review passes from one level to the next. Most institutions take extensive measures to protect the privacy of the candidate by preserving the confidentiality of the information it receives about him or her. At the same time, institutions expect that candidates will similarly respect the confidentiality of the process. Therefore, under normal circumstances, the candidate should not request or seek to discover confidential information from individuals within or outside the home institution who may be involved in the review process. The department chair will be in the best position to address any ambiguities or concerns the candidate might have in this regard.

Promotion Rates

Promotion rates are tracked in various ways. At Stanford University, data for faculty in the tenure line are organized by 5-year hire cohorts with outcomes across four categories (tenured, denied tenure, resigned, or other [including those who were to be reviewed at a future date]). For example, of the 107 tenure-line assistant professors hired into clinical and basic science departments from 1990 to 1999, 65 were granted tenure, 6 were denied tenure, 18 resigned, and 18 fell into other categories, which resulted, for that hire cohort, in a tenure rate of 60.7 %. However, when you isolate the 71 faculty who came up for tenure, the success rate rises to 92 %.

The Association of American Medical Colleges (AAMC) analyzes promotion rates for tenure track and non-tenure-track assistant and associate professors in a similar manner. The data are collected and analyzed through its Faculty Roster database, which is the only national database on the employment, training, and demographic background of US medical school faculty. Findings from this analysis were published in AAMC's Analysis in Brief, which included promotion rates for tenure and non-tenure-track assistant and associate professors, as well as the number of years to promotion (Table 7.2).

Table 7.2 Promotion rates for tenure and non-tenure-track assistant and associate professors and number of years to promotion from AAMC's analysis in brief

| | First-time assistant professors | | | | | | First-time associate professors | | | | | |
| | Average 10-year promotion rates | | | Average no. of years to promotion for promoted faculty | | | Average 10-year promotion rates | | | Average no. of years to promotion for promoted faculty | | |
Study group	1967–1976 Cohorts	1977–1986 Cohorts	1987–1996 Cohorts	1967–1976 Cohorts	1977–1986 Cohorts	1987–1996 Cohorts	1967–1976 Cohorts	1977–1986 Cohorts	1987–1996 Cohorts	1967–1976 Cohorts	1977–1986 Cohorts	1987–1996 Cohorts
All faculty	43.5	40.4	32.8	5.2	5.8	6.2	41.7	42.6	38.6	5.7	5.9	6.1
Clinical departments												
M.D. or Equivalent	44.7	39.4	31.2	5.1	5.8	6.3	44.1	43.1	37.8	5.6	5.9	6.2
Ph.D. or Equivalent	37.9	37.6	30.8	5.6	5.8	6.3	28.9	35.3	33.0	6.0	6.2	6.2
M.D. and Ph.D. or Equivalent	55.0	52.1	48.1	4.9	5.6	6.0	51.2	54.0	49.8	5.6	5.7	5.9
Basic sciences												
M.D. or Equivalent	39.0	37.0	33.2	5.1	5.9	6.2	46.9	43.4	40.1	6.1	5.9	6.0
Ph.D. or Equivalent	54.5	53.9	44.2	5.5	5.8	6.2	42.3	47.1	44.8	5.5	5.6	5.4
M.D. and Ph.D. or Equivalent	44.7	42.0	50.0	5.4	5.5	6.2	44.6	49.7	46.5	5.5	5.6	6.4
Men	44.0	42.6	35.6	5.1	5.7	6.2	42.9	44.2	39.8	5.7	5.9	6.1
Women	36.0	32.1	26.4	5.7	6.2	6.5	31.0	32.6	34.1	6.0	6.2	6.4
White (Not Hispanic/Latino)	46.3	42.6	34.9	5.2	5.8	6.2	42.7	43.9	40.2	5.7	5.9	6.1
Non-white	32.6	30.9	25.2	5.4	5.8	6.3	35.0	36.0	31.1	5.9	6.0	6.2
Tenure track	71.8	51.6	46.8	5.0	5.7	6.2	52.2	51.2	48.6	5.6	5.9	6.0
Non-tenure track	46.4	33.8	28.0	5.4	5.9	6.3	34.5	32.3	29.2	5.5	5.9	6.3

The relatively low promotion rates of 54.9 % for tenure track and 35.2 % for non-tenure-track assistant professors in the 1987–1993 hire cohort were likely influenced, as are the Stanford percentages, by the number of faculty who did not come up for promotion. For example, outcomes for a hire cohort of 120 assistant professors could include 70 faculty who were promoted, 20 faculty who were not promoted, and 30 faculty who, due to resignation or other factors, did not come up for promotion. In looking at the entire cohort, the promotion rate would be 58 %. However, the rate would rise to 78 % for actions in which a promotion decision was rendered. Generally, promotion rates are higher for those groups of faculty who successfully travel through their first and second terms as assistant professors and undergo the promotion review.

Data on national outcomes and trends are helpful to academic leaders in calibrating promotion rates at their own institutions. However, pathways to individual promotion reviews are as varied and unique as the candidates themselves. And outcomes are dependent upon many factors including, importantly, a strong partnership between the candidate and institution on which a successful case for promotion can be made.

Words to the Wise
- Demystify the promotion process by reading the faculty handbook, studying websites, reviewing template letters to referees, and clinical/teaching evaluation forms. Understand policies regarding promotion clock extensions and early promotions.
- Collect and organize contributions cumulatively through an e-portfolio.
- Gather perspectives from mentors and colleagues but identify one person—usually the department chair (or designate)—who will serve as the authoritative interpreter of criteria and of the promotion review process.
- Attend and actively participate in career development and promotion workshops.

(continued)

(continued)

- Meet annually with department chair to track progress toward promotion. Incorporate feedback from midterm review into action plan and refine the timeline that leads to a robust body of scholarship, teaching, and clinical contributions by the time the promotion package is submitted.
- Understand the timing of the promotion review and when candidate materials are due.
- Circulate promotion package to mentors and colleagues for review and advice.
- Determine which, if any, information can be provided post-promotion package submission (e.g., accepted publications, awards, grants).

Ask Your Mentor or Colleagues

- What should you do when the guidance you are receiving from your mentor conflicts with your own sense of what is needed for promotion?
- What was the most important feedback you received from your midterm review?
- How did you find the right voice in writing your candidate's statement for two audiences: experts in your field and faculty from other disciplines?
- What is the most valuable lesson you learned from the promotion process?

Appendix: Sample Promotion Process Timeline

Clock	Tasks
14 months before promotion	Dean's office and department confer about the promotion review
13 months before promotion	Dean's Office sends email notifying the faculty member that the review has commenced, copying the department chair. Faculty member provides CV, candidate's statement, list of current and former trainees, suggested referees, teaching evaluations, and sample publications

Clock	Tasks
12 months before promotion	Department identifies the review committee members. Department reviews candidate's materials and requests revisions, if necessary
11 months before promotion	Department compiles referee list and, if appropriate, the comparison peer list. Department solicits evaluations from internal and external referees and trainees. Department chair makes writing assignments for all sections of the promotion file requiring written text (scholarship, clinical duties, teaching duties, etc.).
10 months before promotion	Department awaits receipt of referee and trainee letters and sends reminders, if necessary
9 months before promotion	Department receives most or all of the referee and trainee letters. Sections on scholarship, clinical and teaching activities are finalized
8 months before promotion	Department receives all referee and trainee letters. All written portions of the file are completed. The review committee has met or a meeting is scheduled. Post-review, the review committee provides a written evaluation of the candidate
7 months before promotion	Department concludes its review by any and all voting bodies. Department completes promotion file. Dean's Office reviews file and suggests revisions, if necessary
6 months before promotion	Final version of the departmental file is prepared for review by higher levels
5 months before promotion	School conducts review. This step may involve multiple levels of review (e.g., Appointments and Promotions Committee, Dean)
1–4 months before promotion	University conducts review. (This step may involve multiple levels of review, e.g., university-wide review committee, Provost, President). Candidate is informed of the promotion decision.
Promotion becomes effective	Formal notification letters are issued. Administrative systems are updated

References

1. Trower CA, Gallagher AS. Perspectives on what pre-tenure faculty want and what six research universities provide. Cambridge, MA: Harvard Graduate School of Education; 2008.
2. JAMA Instructions for Authors. http://jama.ama-assn.org/site/misc/ifora.xhtml#AuthorshipCriteriaandContributionsandAuthorshipForm.

How to Build a National Reputation for Academic Promotion

8

Sidney Zisook and Laura B. Dunn

At most academic institutions, promotion from assistant to associate level in clinical, research, or any other academic track requires the individual to demonstrate that one has developed an outstanding local and regional reputation in an area of expertise. Promotion to professor requires developing an excellent national, if not international, reputation. As there is no single best route to achieving a strong academic reputation, this chapter focuses on principles that help early career academicians to best position themselves to seize and capitalize on opportunities to attain this goal. Obstacles that can impede achievement of a national reputation also are discussed.

Start Early, If You Can

If you don't know where you are going, you might wind up someplace else.

Yogi Berra

When selecting a residency or fellowship, consider not only short-term needs to get excellent clinical training in a program

L.B. Dunn, M.D. (✉)
Department of Psychiatry, University of California, San Francisco,
401 Parnassus Ave., San Francisco, CA, USA
e-mail: laura.dunn@ucsf.edu

© Springer International Publishing Switzerland 2016
109
L.W. Roberts (ed.), *The Associate Professor Guidebook*,
DOI 10.1007/978-3-319-28001-1_8

where residents appear satisfied and respected, but also longer term goals of preparing for an academic career. A resident who aspires to a successful academic career that will, by necessity, require the development of an excellent national reputation would be wise to select a program with faculty members who have attained strong national reputations. Some programs are more successful as launching pads for competitive fellowships or academic appointments. The best way to find out is to ask focused questions of training directors, residents, fellows, and junior faculty at the interviews such as "Do trainees have opportunities, dedicated time, mentorship, and available resources to develop areas of interest most important to them?" "What do residents do after graduation?" "How many go into the most competitive fellowships?" "Where do they go for fellowships?" "How many graduates assume leadership positions in the field and develop national or international reputations?"

For trainees interested in basic, translational, or clinical research, a research-oriented department with top scientists on the faculty bears careful consideration. For the trainee aspiring to develop a reputation as an academic clinician-educator, a program with a clinical scholar or clinical educator track may be especially appealing. For someone who is undecided about post-training plans, a program with a broad range of opportunities and mentors is ideal.

At the faculty level, it may be more difficult to select the ideal program as faculty positions may be more limited. Since the best predictor of the future is the past, it may be wise to visit a program more than once to learn how successful early-career faculty have been in developing their reputations and attaining advancement. Some questions to consider are "Do junior faculty feel satisfied and valued?" "Do they foresee opportunities for advancement?" "Are adequate resources available—including mentorship, time and encouragement to build their academic portfolios and reputations?"

Do your homework to evaluate whether junior faculty have advanced to senior leadership and academic positions, either at the same institution or elsewhere. It is also important to evaluate the degree to which faculty have developed or are developing regional, national, and international reputations. Some questions to consider are "Do junior faculty participate actively in national and international organizations?" "Do they attend meetings of these organizations?" "Do they feel that they have colleagues who are looking out for them?" "Do they have mentors who introduce them to others in the field or otherwise help them to become known?"

Other departmental and institutional factors can affect your ability to develop a national reputation, but such factors may take more investigation. These include the overall functioning and stability of the department and the role of the Chair and other senior leadership. A department without a permanent chair, or one in severe financial difficulty, may not be as conducive for the development of academic faculty. Some Chairs see the development of early-career faculty—introducing them to key players in their field of interest, facilitating invitations to appropriate national organizations, helping with grant applications, protecting them from too much service—as a core feature of their main mission, while others are less focused on or dedicated to faculty development. Therefore, it may be important to know how generative and dedicated to faculty development the Chair and other departmental leaders are when choosing between job offers.

There are several "tracks" available for academic physicians. Navigating each pathway requires knowledge of what is available, the local institutional "culture," and the process and criteria most relevant to the chosen path [1]. The hierarchy of faculty ranks in many academic medical centers include moving up the ladder from Instructor to Assistant Professor to Associate Professor and finally to Professor. In many centers, the qualifiers, "clinical" or "research," or their equivalents, may be attached to the title, for example, Clinical Assistant Professor or Research Professor. Table 8.1 describes a general overview of what promotion committees look for in each major academic "track." For the research scholar, for example, the rank of Research Professor (sometimes just called Professor) is the goal, and promotion is based on a strong national and international reputation in research. To a lesser extent, teaching and possibly even clinical skills may be important. The focus is more on publishing manuscripts and obtaining peer-reviewed funding than it is on seeing patients.

The educator and clinical scholar generally are required to build a strong reputation as a teacher and clinician, and less so as

Table 8.1. Academic tracks

| | | Track | | |
		Research scholar	Clinical scholar/educator	Clinical
Accomplish-ments/ reputation	Example title	Research professor or professor of X	Professor of clinical X	Clinical professor
Research (manuscripts/ grants)		☑☑☑	☑☑	☑
Education/ training		☑☑	☑☑☑	☑☑
Clinical		☑☑	☑☑	☑☑☑

☑☑☑ = strong reputation required for promotion

☑☑ = some accomplishments may be required or desired

☑ = not usually required

an independent investigator. Teaching innovations and creative curricular development may be more important than original research or the number of publications in this track. Finally, the clinician is judged primarily on clinical excellence, often less so on teaching and minimally on research. The sooner you know the idiosyncrasies of each track at your institution, the more likely you are to take the appropriate steps to ensure success in achieving excellent reputations in the field, leading to timely promotions and the satisfaction, prestige and awards that go with them.

Follow Your Passion, Once You Find It

Don't ask what the world needs. Rather ask—what makes you come alive? Then go and do it! Because what the world needs is people who have come alive.

Howard Thurman

Being a physician remains a privileged and honored profession. Few professions offer as many choices—to be a healer, a teacher, a scientist, an expert in medical law, a bioinformatics specialist, to name a few—for a fulfilling and purposeful career. However, it can be challenging to find which among these many possibilities best matches your interests, talents, and temperament. For those who choose careers in academic medicine, the menu can be overwhelming.

While it is important to focus on the areas of academic medicine (e.g., clinical work, teach, research, and community service), it is helpful to understand that whatever early decisions are made, they are not written in stone—people do change directions and adjust their relative emphases on roles over time. It is not unusual for an M.D./Ph.D. to enter a residency fully intent on setting the basic science research world on fire when they graduate, only to find they love caring for patients and to shift to a more clinically oriented career. Similarly, it is not unusual for someone with minimal or no background in research to become excited by the world of discovery during their training and ultimately develop into an outstanding investigator. Thus, early career academicians are faced with the task of discovering their unique academic passions, following them, while being open and flexible to emerging attractions.

Strive for Everyday Excellence

The best preparation for tomorrow is to do today's work superbly well.

William Osler

If there is one *sine qua non* for building a national reputation, it is establishing a local reputation as a reliable colleague and a trustworthy team player who always strives towards excellence. The ACGME competencies provide a useful framework: (1) knowledge (in your general discipline and specific field of concentration), (2) clinical skills (for purposes of professional careers in academic medicine, this can be broadened to include also teaching skills and research skills), (3) practice-based learning and improvement (be at the cutting edge and do what is necessary to stay there), (4) interpersonal and communication skills (in day-to-day work with colleagues, students, and the public as well as in disseminating work verbally and in writing),

(5) professionalism (a commitment to adhering to ethical principles, respect for others, and personal integrity), and (6) systems-based practice (working within the unique intricacies of available resources and the "culture" of your department, university, and national organizations). Attention to each of these areas is much more fruitful than focusing on the more expansive goal of attaining a "national reputation" and is an effective strategy towards academic success.

> *A dream doesn't become reality through magic; it takes sweat, determination and hard work.*
>
> (Colin Powell)

Being an academic physician is hard work. Few academicians begin their careers as fully funded investigators, and no one starts a career as a fully funded teacher or clinician. Thus, academic faculty frequently have several institutional responsibilities and often find themselves with multiple roles including front-line clinical treatment and care. Moreover, faculty often have responsibilities related to patients, students, colleagues, supervisors, mentors, organizations, and communities and to their families. They may be surprised to find themselves working even harder as junior faculty than they did as residents. If they want to make their mark as investigators, they may have to write manuscripts and grant applications in the evenings and on weekends. It may be wise to have frank discussions with your life partner about such demands to make sure that each of you is prepared for the sacrifices. Despite the hard work, when the chair requests a patient to be seen, or your mentor asks for a review of a manuscript he or she has just written, as junior faculty the answer should almost always be, "Happily," or "Of course." For the most part, bargaining and negotiating are skills to use as one moves into mid-career and later.

Say Yes

> *I only have "yes" men around me. Who needs "no" men?*
>
> Mae West

While it is always an asset to be collegial and a good team player, it is especially important early in your career to take advantage of every possible opportunity. The first step in developing a national reputation is developing a local one, and the trainee or early-career faculty member who is viewed as eagerly doing more than his or her share is well on the way. A resident who wants to be nominated for one of the many scholarships, fellowship, travel awards, and other honors available to residents generally does so by being considered a "good citizen" of the residency and department. Personal qualities are every bit as important, sometimes more so, than native intelligence or even accomplishments in getting recognized and promoted. One of the key personal qualities is being considered a giving team player. For both house staff and faculty, the individual who looks at a request more as an opportunity than a burden has an advantage. Even better is the person who does not wait to be asked, but who volunteers for service such as teaching, seeing a difficult patient, serving on committees, consulting to another service, and covering for a colleague in need. Rarely does a promotion committee's recommendation omit "teamwork." Regardless of how much time you lament that too much of your time is spent in front of your computer instead of with patients or students, or that you are too tethered to your cell phone and pager when you would prefer to be free to think, read or, importantly, relax, professionalism demands that you answer pages promptly, return calls, and respond to emails. Part of the reputation you build along the way is directly related to day-to-day communications, electronic or otherwise.

Just Say No (Thanks)

It comes from saying no to 1,000 things to make sure we don't get on the wrong track or try to do too much. We're always thinking about new markets we could enter, but it's only by saying no that you can concentrate on the things that are really important.

Steve Jobs

There comes a time when "Yes, thank you; more, please" cannot remain the default reply to all requests. No one can do it all, which often requires learning the art of saying "No, thank you." To protect your time and to focus on unique academic passions and career goals, it becomes important to recognize limits and eliminate extraneous pursuits. Books have been written on the gentle art of saying no [2]. Usually a straightforward "Thanks for the offer, but I just have too much on my plate right now" will do. There is no reason to apologize for not being a super hero; none of us are. If someone such as a Chair, the Dean or another important "boss" is asking, and especially if he is insistent, it sometimes helps to review with them other commitments and enlist their help in re-prioritizing. You may be able to reach a compromise, and an initial "No, thank you" may turn into "Can I get back to you in a few weeks? or, I'll try to get to it next month." But sometimes, it is incumbent on the individual to respect his or her own priorities and time (for more on "saying no" see Chap. 15).

Find the Right Mentor

A self-taught man usually has a poor teacher and a worse student.

Henny Youngman

The right mentor can help pave the road to an outstanding reputation in many ways. The prime responsibility of a mentor is to help guide the mentee to a rewarding and successful career in academic medicine [3]. Research has found that mentorship in academic medicine has an important influence on personal development and productivity [4], perhaps especially for women [5] and minorities [6]. Mentorship can take many forms. For the research scientist, this may entail help in developing a research focus, finding grant support, publishing, and presenting findings. Mentors can also help the up-and-coming researcher find ongoing projects to get involved in or datasets to mine while they wait for their own research to be funded or to begin yielding results.

For the educator, a mentor may focus on helping the mentee develop teaching skills and finding opportunities to teach both locally and to broader audiences. Mentors also assist mentees in getting involved in curriculum development, presenting their creative ideas in other settings outside the department and university, and navigating the institutional system to find teaching and administrative positions in the medical school or department.

For the clinical scholar, a mentor might help the mentee learn to turn a clinical conundrum into a researchable question or literature review, and a challenging patient into a publishable case report. Effective mentors are also good role models. They help their mentees learn when to say "Yes" and when to decline. They may also provide advice on difficult topics such as balancing work, family, leisure, and health. An important role mentors have is advocating for and promoting their mentees in the department, medical school, and national organizations. An effective mentor often introduces mentees to other potential mentors, supervisors, and collaborators. Often multiple mentors may provide complimentary roles. Perhaps most important, mentors provide guidance on what it takes to develop an outstanding reputation and get promoted.

Sign Up

I don't know what your destiny will be, but one thing I know: the only ones among you who will be really happy are those who have sought and found how to serve.

Albert Schweitzer

Initiating, sustaining, and nurturing connections with others, referred to as "networking," generally require active participation in local and national conferences and organizations. Be proactive. Awards, fellowships, and scholarships are available for residents, fellows, junior residents, and junior faculty. Do not assume that just because your training director, mentor, or chair has not nominated you that you are not competitive, or even that they know what is out there. Ask. If they do not know, ask other faculty members from inside and outside your department, colleagues, and acquaintances from other programs. Be creative about searching for awards and fellowships, check society websites and the NIH website. When you hear about awards or fellowships, let your immediate supervisors know of your interest.

At meetings, it is useful to seek out established investigators and "experts" and introduce yourself to let them know of your interest in their work. Junior scholars are often surprised at how accessible the academic "superstars" are, and how willing they are to offer advice and guidance. When possible, mentors can play an important role in making introductions and facilitating these connections. A second way to meet established academicians is to present a talk or poster at national conferences. Some of the most interesting and intense discussions occur during poster sessions–often more so than during more formal presentations or talks. A third way is to participate in workshops and symposia. Not only does this give the presenter a chance to disseminate her work, it also fosters connections with other investigators. Also, take the initiative to organize and submit a symposium, asking established experts to join can be a great way to be seen as a leader and to build long-lasting relationships.

Fellowships and Training Grants

> Training is everything. The peach was once a bitter almond; cauliflower is nothing but cabbage with a college education.
>
> Mark Twain

While clinical positions are often available immediately after residencies, an important intermediary step for the budding research scholars is a research fellowship. The "right" fellowship provides training in necessary research skills and mentorship regarding academic and general career development. It provides you with time to build your CV, attain research support before applying for academic appointments, and obtain opportunities to network to further develop your academic reputation. There a variety of postdoctoral research training programs available to residency training graduates [7]. Among them, NIH funded institutional T32 Training Grants (http://grants.nih.gov/training/nrsa.htm) providing stipends and an institutional allowance, are specifically designed to provide young scientists with experience in research methodology and to train the next generation of physician scholars. Often, one of the key goals in T32 or other research fellowships is for the young investigator to emerge with research funding, such as a K award. The NIH career development (K series) is a key vehicle for successful progression to independent investigator (http://grants.nih.gov/training/careerdevelopmenta-wards.htm). A K award validates for the candidate, professional colleagues, and the funding agency that the recipient has made a serious commitment to life as a researcher [8]. These typically provide a much higher level of salary support than other research grants and require at least a 75 % time commitment, which allows junior investigators the necessary protected time to develop their own research programs.

Write

Either write something worth reading or do something worth writing.
Benjamin Franklin

For many academic physicians, manuscripts and grants are the key currencies for promotion, for building a reputation, and for disseminating creative accomplishments. For clinical scholars and research scientists, the quality and quantity of peer-reviewed manuscripts are important components of building a reputation and at least some of the publications should be in high impact journals. In the earliest stages, contributing to manuscripts, even in a limited way in multi-authored papers, represents a good start, but eventually some first authored papers are necessary, both for promotion and for building a reputation. Sometimes, only the first author is remembered. Later in your career, being last, or "senior" author conveys even more status than first authorship, as it communicates being the "leader of the team."

Embrace Failure

I've failed over and over and over again in my life and that is why I succeed.

Michael Jordan

Success consists of going from failure to failure without loss of enthusiasm.

Winston Churchill

There is no way to succeed in academics without taking risks. When submitting a paper for publication, it is often wise to aim for a journal that is more widely read, or more academically prestigious, than where you think it is likely to get accepted. For one thing, you never know and for another you often receive feedback to improve the quality of the work. It can be the equivalent of free expert supervisory or mentor advice. Requests for revision or even frank rejections must be seen as opportunities to do better rather than personal criticisms. Most reviewers do not feel they are doing jobs if they just praise a submission or accept it outright, therefore, even the most established academicians rarely receive immediate acceptances on their initial submissions. This is even truer of grant applications, where the vast majority of submissions never get funded and those that do achieve funding often do so only after one or two revised applications. Trying may mean that you may sometimes fail but, more importantly, that you will also sometimes succeed.

Words to the Wise
- Strive for excellence, not for reputation.
- Be known as a good friend, classmate, and colleague first and foremost.
- Learn to focus on what is most important to one's academic passions and values, even if it means sometimes saying "no."
- Publish—often and well.
- Network.
- Volunteer.
- Collaborate.
- Reach out to others, including to faculty more junior than you and to the public.

Ask Your Mentor or Colleagues
- What do I need to do here to succeed?
- What is most likely to derail me from developing a national reputation? How can I best avoid those roadblocks? Are there examples of either you can share with me?

(continued)

(continued)

- How do I ensure time to write and for my own research (or teaching)?
- Who should I get to know here? Locally? Nationally? Internationally? Can you help me meet them? If not you, who?
- What organizations should I join?
- What awards, scholarships, and fellowships are available for me?
- How important is it for me to review manuscripts? Research proposals? If important, can you help me let people know I am available?

References

1. Buchanan GR. Academic promotion and tenure: a user's guide for junior faculty members. Am Soc Hematol. 2009;2009:736–41.
2. Grzyb JE, Chandler R. The nice factor: the art of saying no. London: Fusion; 2008.
3. Jotkowitz A, Clarfield M. Mentoring in internal medicine. Eur J Intern Med. 2006;17:399–401.
4. Sambunjak D, Straus SE, Marusić A. Mentoring in academic medicine. J Am Med Assoc. 2006;296: 1103–15.
5. McGuire LK, Bergen MR, Polan ML. Career advancement for women faculty in a U.S. school of medicine: perceived needs. Acad Med. 2004;79:319–25.
6. Benson CA, Morahan PS, Sachdeva AK, Richman RC. Effective faculty preceptoring and mentoring during reorganization of an academic medical center. Med Teach. 2002;7:717–24.
7. Podskalny JM. NIH early career funding opportunities. Gastroenterology. 2011;141:1159–962.
8. Kupfer DJ, Schatzberg AF, Grochocinski VJ, Dunn LO, Kelley KA, O'Hara RM. The Career Development Institute for Psychiatry: an innovative, longitudinal program for physician-scientists. Acad Psychiatry. 2009;33(4):313–8.

How to "Pitch" a Nontraditional Career Path

9

Margaret S. Chisolm

Understanding how to turn a nontraditional journey to academic medicine into an asset rather than a liability is essential to academic success and eventual promotion. As you reflect on who you are and where you have been, you will gain insights to guide you closer toward your destination. By claiming your expertise and leveraging your assets as you design a strategy for the future, you will ensure that the time and energy spent on your nontraditional path has not been wasted. Being a curious and observant person will allow you to identify urgent problems and leverage your unique background to come up with innovative solutions. With the support of your institution and department, if you stay focused and are able to clearly communicate the impact of your work, you will achieve success. Your nontraditional path toward academic medicine has the potential not only to bring you promotion but also to make a unique impact on your institution, department, colleagues, students, patients, and the communities you serve.

M.S. Chisolm, M.D. (✉)
Department of Psychiatry and Behavioral Sciences, Johns Hopkins University, 5300 Alpha Commons Drive, Baltimore, MD, USA
e-mail: mchisoll@jhmi.edu

© Springer International Publishing Switzerland 2016
L.W. Roberts (ed.), *The Associate Professor Guidebook*,
DOI 10.1007/978-3-319-28001-1_9

Defining a Nontraditional Career Path

Students arrive at medical school via a range of paths, both traditional and nontraditional. Nontraditional medical students might come to medical school following a postbaccalaureate pre-medicine program entered right after college or might come to medical school after a long career in an entirely different field. Once in medical school, these nontraditional students blend with those students fresh from college. Some medical students from both groups—nontraditional and traditional backgrounds—will end up pursuing academic careers.

Physicians also develop academic careers via a range of traditional and nontraditional paths. This chapter focuses on those individuals who came to academic medicine via the "road less traveled." Rather than joining an academic medicine department as a resident or fellow directly after residency, these individuals chose to start a practice in the community, to join a nonacademic hospital practice, to work outside the home part-time or not at all, or to pursue an array of individual passions. And now—for whatever reason—they find themselves returning to an academic medicine environment. If you are one of these physicians, coming back to an academic program, welcome! This chapter is for you.

During the time you spent outside academic medicine, you have accumulated a body of knowledge, experiences, and skills that are unique to you and distinct from those who have followed more traditional academic paths. This chapter will discuss how best to push off from a nontraditional foundation to most efficiently reach the three markers of academic success: (1) focused productivity, (2) scholarly impact, and (3) nationally- and internationally-recognized expertise.

Know Thyself

Before getting started, your first task will be to take a self-inventory. What do you know and what do you do best? Since you are the person most invested in your academic success, you will need to assess your strengths honestly. Psychiatrists are trained to assess the temperamental strengths and vulnerabilities of their patients. So, if you are a psychiatrist, this step may come more easily to you than to those trained in other medical specialties. Regardless of your background, if you have not already formally assessed your own temperament via the NEO-PI or Meyers-Briggs Type Indicator, now is the time to do it. A free Keirsey Temperament Sorter [1], based on the Meyers-Briggs, will help you assess your interests, the kind of data to which you pay attention, how you make decisions, and how you prefer to live your life—all of which can provide insight into your own innate attitudes.

Knowing your temperament will help you gauge how best to manage your time so as to achieve focused productivity. It will also help you answer questions like "Do you enjoy working on your own or in groups?" "Are you by nature detail-oriented or are you more of a 'big picture' person?" "Do you prefer working with objective data or are you more comfortable in the subjective realm of meaning?" "Are you able to set your own goals and easily remain focused on the task at hand or do you need more external structure to prevent your curiosity and flexibility to stay focused?" Since you will need to manage your time well to be a successful academic, knowing what energizes you, how attentive you are to details, what kind of data you like to work with, and how organized and focused you are will be essential for you to make up for "lost" time and efficiently make your own unique scholarly contribution.

Claim Your Expertise

In addition to getting to know yourself, you will need to take an inventory of the knowledge, experiences, and skills you acquired during your unique nontraditional journey to academic medicine. To make an impact in medicine and in the world, you must first think carefully and expansively about what you have learned, and why it matters. The experiences and the achievements you had while away from academic medicine has value and is credible. But, you first need to claim this expertise—to "own" it—before you build on it to become a recognized expert in this area.

The OpEd Project [2]—an organization with the short-term goal of increasing the number of women thought leaders—asks its participants "Do you understand your knowledge and experience in terms of its value to others?" Put more simply "What do you know?" and "Why does it matter?" These core questions are relevant to anyone who has taken a nontraditional career path and is vulnerable, in an academic setting, to feeling underestimated or devalued. Because you are the person most invested in your academic success, it will be up to you to believe in and communicate the value and credibility of your experiences to others. You need to clearly articulate what you know and why it matters.

Leverage Your Assets

Once you know who you are, what you know, and what you do best—and are able to communicate this to others—you need to start thinking about how you are going to leverage those unique assets most effectively. You need to start thinking strategically about how you are going to demonstrate why and how you are needed. A strategy based on the quality that already distinguishes you from the rest of the faculty members, i.e., your nontraditional career path, is the place to start.

When everyone else zigged, you zagged and you can make that difference work to your advantage. In fact, one of "The 100 Best Business Books of All Time" [3]—*Zag* [4]—suggests this exact strategy as a way for businesses "to separate the winners from the clutter… When everybody zigs, zag." You might ask why an academic physician would look to the business world for career tips, but when you think about the three markers of academic success (focused productivity, impact, and recognition), they seem remarkably similar to those of a successful business brand. In developing a brand, *Zag* suggests you first find what makes you different (your "zag") and then "brand" it by asking yourself questions like: "Where do I have the most credibility?" "Where do I have the most experience?" and "Where does your passion lie?" Or as Laura Roberts asks, "What is it that you cannot *not* do?" Sound familiar? They should, because these questions are part of those first steps of knowing thyself and claiming your expertise. Next, you will need to build on those assets by developing a unique vision.

Create an Innovative Vision

Our Iceberg is Melting: Changing and Succeeding Under Any Conditions [5] is a fable about a penguin colony in Antarctica. The colony has survived for centuries by relying on various traditions. One day, a particularly curious penguin notices a problem that threatens the entire colony's continued existence. Not only does this observant penguin see the problem and recognize its gravity, he also imagines a creative solution to avert the colony's annihilation. But, when he tries to tell the others, they not only doubt the magnitude of the problem but also resist his innovative plan for survival. The fable proceeds to show the series of tactics this lone penguin uses to persuade the rest of the colony to recognize the gravity of the problem and accept his clever solution. You may now be thinking, "Nice penguin story, but what exactly does this have to do with my promotion?"

First, the alarmed penguin is different from the other members of the penguin colony. For the penguin, it his observant and open nature that distinguishes him from his peers; for you, it is your nontraditional background. Second, the penguin has a vision for action that, if implemented, has the potential to make a huge impact on the colony. Likewise, your academic vision should have the potential for societal impact. Third, the penguin needs to persuade others in his colony of the potential impact of his vision just as your ultimate challenge will be to persuade the promotions committee of the impact of your academic work. As you prepare for "pitching" your nontraditional career path to your more traditional colleagues on the promotions committee, you can use the penguin as a model such that you create an innovative vision and develop a strategy that builds on your assets (who you are, what you know, and what you do best).

As part of an overall strategy for achieving impact and recognition in your area of credibility, experience, and passion, both *Zag* and *Our Iceberg is Melting* recommend being focused and productive in an area of innovation. *Zag* offers relevant strategies such as spotting a trend (think NIH funding priorities or new clinical or educational needs) and "riding" it. *Our Iceberg is Melting* stresses the need to be curious and observant. Then, when a problem or need is identified, *Iceberg* says you need to come up with a vision and strategy to solve the problem. Being able to see what is possible and work in an innovative area is a smart strategy for those with a nontraditional career path who are making up for "lost time." Being one of the first to focus on a particular problem will enable you to become a respected expert most efficiently. If, instead, you stay with the herd and pursue what others are already doing, it will take longer to become a recognized thought leader. Coupled with a guiding team of mentors to ensure you are being systematic and careful enough, I would suggest being as fearless as the fabled penguin in creating your vision and strategy.

Stay Focused

Although you always need to remain open to the world of possibilities around you, you ultimately also need to be focused and productive. The need for focus cannot be stressed enough. Academic medicine is an intellectually stimulating environment. It is filled with interesting ideas, opportunities, and people. That is why you have chosen an academic career. Once you have defined your area of innovation, you need to stick to it. You have a lot of work to do. Do not get distracted by too many other great ideas and opportunities. And although relationships will be important to your academic success via advice and guidance, mentorship, job opportunities, networking, and collaboration [6], you cannot spend all your time socializing. Remember, there is work to be done. You cannot let up. Losing focus represents the biggest threat to your academic success. Stay focused!

Tell a Good Story

In addition to claiming and leveraging your expertise, creating your innovative vision, and staying focused you will need to become an expert communicator if you want to be productive as a scholar and to "pitch" your nontraditional career path. *The OpEd Project* goal is to have more women thought leaders represented in newspapers' opinion and editorial pages. Like *Zag*, which walks its readers through the steps necessary to articulate a purpose and vision, *The OpEd Project* demands its participants claim their expertise and persuasively present an idea about which they are passionate. Through this process, participants hone their verbal and written communication skills, and so develop into engaging and persuasive op-ed writers. The OpEd Project motto is "Whoever tells the story writes history!"

Likewise, *Our Iceberg is Melting* teaches you, the reader, to share your story—what is your vision and how will you get there—in a way that is focused, attention-grabbing, concrete, and credible. Choosing your language carefully so that others can see the impact of your work is important not only to writing grants and getting your message out via talks and publications, but is crucial to academic promotion. You need to believe in and advocate for yourself. Communicating is your main way of advocating for yourself. You need to tell your story.

Sit at the Table

As Facebook COO Sheryl Sandberg says, "Sit at the table!!" [7] Just make sure you are sitting at the right table—the adults' table, not the kids' table. To help you leverage your expertise in a focused and productive way, you will need to develop a "power base" of supporters—chairs, senior faculty, and mentors—who buy into your vision and will advocate for your success. It will pay to develop professional relationships with each member of this support team, not only so they can get to know your work, but also so that they can get to know you. Each person will need to respect your strengths and not try to make you into someone you are not. The members of this support team will need to believe in the impactful innovation of your work and in your ability to communicate this to others. So select your institution, department, and mentors well. If you do not find the support you need from your team, consider other options either inside or outside your institution and department. You will need a respectful and loyal team of leaders to help you leverage your strengths and navigate the academic system. This type of team can provide financial support, time, networking opportunities, and moral support to help you get through some difficult waters. However, the team members need to believe in you and make a place for you at the table.

To sit at the table, you will have to "put on the suit"—literally. In your nontraditional career, you may have been able to come to work in a sweater and slacks, or even a bathrobe and slippers. But, academic medical leaders wear suits. Like it or not, the right clothing will help give you the credibility you need for promotion and you will need to put on the suit. If you are in doubt about your wardrobe, you may consider seeking out a trusted senior faculty member to tell you whether or not you are dressing professionally. Be observant of your surroundings and look at what individuals in leadership positions wear at your institution. You may also want to read books on how to dress for success. You may even benefit from working with a professional image consultant. The right clothing is not going to ensure your academic success, but the wrong clothing—especially for women, short men, and minorities—can jeopardize your place at the table [8].

Conclusion

Good leaders know that everyone will benefit from your success. You, as an individual, have unique strengths. Your nontraditional background confers a different set of knowledge, experiences, and skills than more traditional colleagues. If you claim your expertise and leverage it to create an innovative, focused, and productive body of scholarship, everyone will benefit. Your work will enrich not only you and your institution, your department, and your faculty and learners but—ultimately—patients and families. To be sure, some institutions, departments, and leaders will not recognize, acknowledge, or respect your strengths as having a place in academic medicine. But, although some may not see a role for individuals with nontraditional career paths in academic medicine, diversity—including the diversity that comes from having a faculty that includes individuals with nontraditional backgrounds—increases innovation and creativity. Your nontraditional path has the potential to bring you scholarly recognition and allow you to make a unique impact.

Words to the Wise
- Know thyself
- Claim your expertise
- Leverage your assets
- Create an innovative vision
- Stay focused
- Tell a good story
- Sit at the table
- And know that everyone benefits from diversity

Ask Your Mentor or Colleagues
- What is your perspective on the strengths and vulnerabilities of my temperament?
- What knowledge, experience, and skills distinguish me favorably from my peers?
- How do you think I can best leverage my assets in the institution and department?
- Do you see an opportunity for innovation in an area within my expertise? If so, who are the thought leaders in this area, locally, nationally, and internationally? How might I get to know them (e.g., organizational committees, journal reviews, collaborations)? Can you introduce me?
- Are there any key leaders in the institution and department who I should get to know? If so, are there tangible ways in which I could get to know them (e.g., shared committees, courses, collaborations)? Can you introduce me?

References

1. Personality test based on Jung and Briggs Myers typology. http://www.humanmetrics.com/cgi-win/JTypes2.asp. Accessed 12 Dec 2011.
2. Welcome to the Op-Ed Project. http://www.theopedproject.org. Accessed 12 Dec 2011.

3. The 100 Best Business Books of All Time. http://www.100bestbiz.com. Accessed 12 Dec 2011.
4. Neumeier M. Zag: the number-one strategy of high-performance brands. Berkeley, CA: New Riders; 2007.
5. Kotter J, Rathgeber H. Our iceberg is melting: changing and succeeding under any condition. New York, NY: St. Martin's Press; 2005.
6. Chisolm M. Transitioning to academic medicine while maintaining balance: working harder, not smarter. Acad Med. 2011;35(3):165–7.
7. Sheryl Sandberg: why we have too few women leaders. http://www.ted.com/talks/sheryl_sandberg_why_we_have_too_few_women_leaders.html. Accessed 12 Dec 2011.
8. Molloy J. New women's dress for success. New York, NY: Business Plus; 1996. p. 7.

How to Be an Effective Team Leader and Committee Member or Chair

10

Sabine C. Girod

Academic leaders are often chosen based on their academic success and reputation in the core mission of research over teaching and patient care. However, leadership of a team, committee, or department in an Academic Medical Center (AMC) also requires knowledge of clinical operations and finances, as well as administrative and managerial skills that are usually not part of the academic medical education or career. Many AMCs have recognized the need for effective physician leaders to successfully advance innovation and improve the clinical care of patients. They offer educational programs to help their faculty grow into leadership roles spanning the traditional silos of hospital administration, clinical care, research, and education of the next generation of physicians and scientists. The academic physician is encouraged to take advantage of these opportunities. The skills one will learn will greatly benefit one's academic career even if one does not choose a traditional leadership position.

What are the skills that make a good academic leader? While successful leaders have widely differing backgrounds and personality traits, they generally excel in vision, communication, and strategic planning. The special challenge to leaders in AMCs is the

S.C. Girod, M.D., D.D.S., Ph.D., F.A.C.S. (✉)
Department of Surgery (Oral Medicine & Maxillofacial Surgery),
Stanford School of Medicine, 770 Welch Road, Suite 400,
Stanford, CA, USA
e-mail: sgirod@stanford.edu

© Springer International Publishing Switzerland 2016   133
L.W. Roberts (ed.), *The Associate Professor Guidebook*,
DOI 10.1007/978-3-319-28001-1_10

different missions and parallel reporting structures, from clinical operations to faculty development, that require the mastery of a range of different leadership styles adapted to the environment. While support staff in a clinic may respond to a more authoritative leadership approach, faculty physicians are independent experts who can only be engaged by means of a democratic communication and decision processes. Academic leaders usually cannot and should not try to employ corporate reward and punishment powers, but need to rely on their interpersonal and persuasive skills to motivate their peers and staff. Participation in academic and administrative committees is usually voluntary for faculty and an opportunity to become engaged in the leadership decision process of their AMC at multiple levels. Faculty can help produce a superior outcome by contributing their expertise and creativity to the leadership of an AMC. In order to fully engage them, leaders need to make faculty team members feel respected and valued for their work.

The Three Pillars of Leadership: Vision, Communication, Organization

Most of us see leadership as a person in power who pulls people in the right direction using a set of acquirable tools. This perception is widely advertised in an infinite number of publications and courses. However, while it is important to learn excellent communication and organizational skills to be a good leader—think of how your clinical skills evolved since medical school to become a good doctor—it does not guarantee leadership success. Leadership is all about understanding and transforming people and their minds and behavior to create change—including and foremost yourself. Your personal integrity and shared values are what other people will respond to, not the leadership tools.

Vision

Before you start working with a group, stop and think about the vision. Where will your division, department, school be in the future? How does the work of your committee fit into an existing vision? A compelling vision has power. It can inspire, clarify, focus, and motivate faculty, students, and/or staff. Draw on the specific strengths of your organization, and create a positive and inspiring statement describing where you want to be in the future, such as "To be the medical school that sets the standard for *educating* physicians, scientists, and teachers to be leaders of change in creating a healthier, better world" (Dartmouth Medical School). Then define the immediate mission of your group's or committee's work in the context of the vision, and determine the milestones that you all will accomplish to reach them. Besides the overall mission and vision, leading a department or committee will of course also involve multiple short-term operational objectives, such as hiring and space, that need to be addressed on an ongoing basis.

Strategic Planning

There are two principal processes how you can develop a vision and mission statement and move forward with your organization. You can either develop the vision yourself and then get "buy-in" from your group or employ a strategic planning process with your group to create the vision and mission statements. In an academic environment, the strategic planning approach is preferable since it is an open, deliberate decision process that focuses the collective vision and expertise of the participants on creating a roadmap for the future. One of the major advantages in an academic environment is that it creates the "buy-in" from the participants whose voices are heard in the process and unites them behind the goal. The process is thus far more important than the plan itself.

Expertise

In order to develop a vision, formulate a mission and successfully lead a committee or department; knowledge of applicable subject matters is essential for leaders and members alike. For a committee, it may be one single subject, while for leadership of a department or division understanding of a wide variety of topics from residency programs to clinical care, reimbursement may be required. While extensive expertise or the access to it is essential for some areas, e.g., finances of a division, others may need less. You will need to make decisions in which areas you will get more involved at what to delegate to others.

Take into account how your activities are perceived by the members of your department or committee. What do they expect and how does your action relate to their core expectations, activities, and values? For example, a leader of a clinical division or medical school should still participate in clinical activities and teaching. It signals to your faculty and staff that you value their work, and it is an excellent way to share and understand their experiences, which will give you better guidance in decision-making processes. A committee leader or member should have expertise and interest in the task the committee is charged with to be able to make meaningful contributions.

One of the most significant expertise necessary for a leader is his or her organizational knowledge, not only the knowledge of the obvious organizational structure but more importantly the inner workings, i.e., politics. Without a good understanding of the personalities and their mission and standing within an organization, it is impossible to lead an academic department.

Risk Taking

Transformative leaders are pioneers who innovate and inspire. Thinking big and outside the box and to reach big goals often requires risk taking. It means taking calculated steps into unknown territory beyond our immediate expertise and comfort zone to find new paths that bring us closer to our goal. If you do not feel comfortable making big decisions, consider taking a planned stepwise approach to create change:

- *P*lan: Identify the problem.
- *D*o: Make a change on a small, experimental scale.
- *C*heck: Have the objectives been achieved?
- *A*ct: If successful, implement changes on a larger scale.

Based on the actions taken, it is called a PDCA cycle and can be repeated until you reach your goal. In the meantime, learn from your failures and become more and more "comfortable with the uncomfortable."

Communication

Outstanding interpersonal skills and communication are the hallmarks of inspiring leaders and members of successful teams. When we think about communication, we almost inevitably associate how we actively speak to others. However, listening effectively is the most important skill for everyone. You need to be aware of other people's motivations, interests, thoughts, and feelings. In direct conversations, it helps to paraphrase what somebody is telling you, both to clarify the meaning for yourself and to signal your interest in what the other person is saying. Understanding people is the prerequisite for effective communication of information, providing feedback and communicating your point of view or vision. All academic faculty know from their teaching experience that the better you know your audience, the better you can address them and get them excited about what you are saying.

Besides the verbal and nonverbal aspects of communication, such as clarity of speaking, eye contact, and body language, communication is about sharing and promoting your values and ideas. If there is no congruence between your values, body language, and what you say verbally, others will inevitably sense insincerity and be wary of you. Again, mastering the tools of communication will not be helpful if your personal self and thinking are not aligned. So be aware of your values, act responsibly, and be accountable. People will judge you by whether your actions follow your communication. If you make a promise, keep it; if you cannot, let the person know immediately. If you do not listen or communicate integrity and reliability in basic interactions, others will not follow and support your grander visions.

Communicating respect and support can create loyalty and support in turn for you as a thought leader in any group—whether you are the appointed leader or the member of a committee or department. Simply thanking and praising others for work well done cannot be overrated. Also never claim all good news for yourself, especially if you are the chair or chief of a department. Let others shine and be the cheerleader for them. They will be more open to your ideas and leadership since they can trust you to recognize their accomplishments and support them. The opposite is true, if you do not listen or even try to compete with your faculty and claim their successes for yourself. Ignored emotions and sensitivities of others due to lack of communication and recognition can be the most significant barriers to your success.

If you are trusted and an expert, people will come to you and ask your advice, and you will probably do the same with your trusted advisors. Access to a network of colleagues or mentors who can be called on for their expertise is most important for your success as an academic faculty and leader. You can get open feedback and reflect your ideas and plans to improve your overall performance.

Organization

Organizational Knowledge and Skills

Planning and organizational skills are necessary to lead all organizations, big or small. AMCs are particularly complex in their organizational structure since the different missions of teaching, clinical work, and research may be run in parallel administrative silos with separate command structures and complex interactions at different levels. For example, the clinical care organization, i.e., hospital, may be run by the school or be a separate entity and as such can be a part of a larger organizational structure. The academic faculty physicians can be part of a hospital physician group, but the reporting structure lies within the academic department. Staff may be part of a department or the hospital and reporting to either, even though they are physically working in the same space. In such complex organizational structures, it can be very difficult to create seamless operations or adapt to a change.

First of all, an excellent knowledge of the particular organizational structures in your AMC is essential. You will probably recognize that much of the influence and power you can exercise depends on your communication skills, since many of the people you are working with belong to a different reporting structure or will not be susceptible to a directive approach, e.g., faculty. As an academic department chief or chair, you will likely have a small core staff that needs to be carefully chosen with regard to excellence in their field of expertise and also their communication skills since they are in a similar situation and will have to negotiate with their peers, e.g., in the hospital administration.

As we already discussed earlier, you will need to decide which areas of your administrative function you will delegate and assess the resources that are necessary, e.g., to run the residency programs, faculty development, and department finances. Similarly, as a committee chair, you need to discuss with your committee members what the tasks are and how the members can contribute individually. Delegation of power or better empowerment of your staff and colleagues is probably the most important task you have to fulfill.

Decision Making

Your task as a leader is in many ways defined by constant decision making, sometimes under pressure. You should review your process and be open to analyzing not only your successes but also your failures. It often helps to have a structured approach that includes definition of the problem, assessment of the implications, exploring perspectives, advantages and disadvantages, and getting clear on what the ideal outcome would be. For more complex decisions, this can take the form of a strategic planning, as discussed above. Getting input from the people affected by the decision, mentors, and peers in your network will help you to develop a better picture of the ramifications of your decision. Once you consider a decision, make sure to communicate it to all involved and get them on board. Understand when your decision has outcomes that are not acceptable to others and would lay the groundwork to continued and possibly widespread discontent in your group. The most important skill is to know when to follow instead of trying to lead.

Effective Meetings

Leadership of an academic department or committee also comes with the responsibility to master the basic principles of running effective meetings. In the case of committees, it starts with the crucial selection of qualified members. It is usually helpful to have a first "kick-off" meeting to determine the meeting time and frequency and discuss the purpose of the meeting. An agenda needs to be prepared for every meeting and circulated to the members beforehand. Everyone appreciates if meetings start and end on time and follows the agenda. More formal deliberations should be conducted according to Robert's Rules of Order (newly revised). Minutes of the meeting including attendance should be recorded by a staff or committee member and approved by the committee.

Do not dominate the meeting if you are a leader or member, but, rather, encourage or contribute ideas and suggestions while moving the agenda along in a timely fashion. Update the members on news relevant to the committee work. Avoid arguments and encourage positive thinking. Any new items should be specified in the agenda and pertinent material be sent out before the meeting. If you need more time or an issue needs to be addressed on a long-term or short-term basis, initiate standing or ad hoc subcommittees who can work on these issues and report back to the committee.

Leadership Styles

No single leadership style fits every situation. To be a good leader, you have to know your group and your preferred leadership style and be able to adapt your style to the changes in your group. Above all, you have to inspire and motivate your team or committee members to change expectations, perceptions, and motivations to work successfully towards a common goal.

Leadership styles have been described among others as *autocratic* (high level of power over group), *charismatic* (encouragement and enthusiasm, power rests with leader), *bureaucratic* (principled, all initiative from leader), *participatory* (teamwork, only leader knows the task), *transactional* ("carrot and cane" approach), and *transformational* (values team members for their individual potential, leads by example). It is generally believed today that transformational leadership is most effective. Transformational leaders communicate their vision and inspire their team to share the vision. They care for the team members more than for the task at hand and modify the communication style depending on the needs and strength of the individual team member to engage him or her and delegate tasks. The major difference to all other styles of leadership is that it takes into account that every person requires a different kind of leadership and communication to be fully engaged in work of the group or committee.

Situational Leadership

Different theories have been developed through research on effective leadership with groups and organizations to provide guidelines for optimal leadership styles in various environments. One of these frameworks is "situational leadership" that is based on the attitude and readiness of the group for a specific task. This theory provides a suitable framework for AMCs, where committees and organizational structures are built around a specific task or mission and either include members from very diverse backgrounds, e.g., administrators, nursing staff, and physicians, or are highly homogenous, e.g., a faculty search committee.

Hersey and Blanchard [1] recommend four different "optimal" leadership styles based on the assessment of the "willingness and ability" of the group:

S1: Telling (unable, insecure)
S2: Selling (unable, willing)
S3: Participating/supporting (capable, unwilling)
S4: Delegating (very capable, confident)

Essentially, the model recommends taking a very directed managerial approach in S1 and a more communicative "selling" approach in S2 to get the members or the group on board. S3 and S4 leadership should be focused on coaching and/or supporting the group members as needed in a participative and transformational leadership model.

Words to the Wise
- Listen and understand the values and motivations of other people.
- Be true to your values and promises at all times.
- Know when to follow and when to lead.
- Lead by example.
- Review successes and failures.
- Reassess your goals and aspirations.

Ask Your Mentor or Colleagues
- What is your favorite leadership style?
- What leaders have influenced you in developing your leadership style?
- How do you select committee members?

Appendix: Examples of Leadership Styles

S2 Scenario

Imagine you are the director of your outpatient clinic and you are trying to improve patient satisfaction by educating your staff to use a programmatic approach to engaging with your patients that makes them feel welcomed and valued. The staff in your clinic is very willing to participate, but they do not seem to have the skills to do it. You communicate the value of the new program and coach and engage staff individually by observation and directed positive feedback until they are comfortable with the new protocol.

S4 Scenario

You are the new chief of an academic division and you are trying to increase the faculty attendance in the faculty meetings and grand rounds. In order to do this, you develop a plan that penalizes the faculty financially on a sliding scale if they do not come to the meetings. They have to sign in to prove that they attended. You present your plan at the next faculty meeting and implement it the following week.

The result? All faculty members resent your plan. They come to the meetings and sign in, but many leave immediately. You have damaged the relationship with your faculty by using an S1 leadership approach to an S4 situation.

Reference

1. Hersey P, Blanchard KH. Management of organizational behavior: utilizing human resources. 3rd ed. New Jersey: Prentice Hall; 1977.

How to Collaborate Interprofessionally

11

Nathan Hantke and Penelope Zeifert

Collaborating with other professionals is not only necessary, but it can also be one of the most rewarding aspects of working within the medical field. Increasingly, medical decisions are being made based upon the input of a team of health care providers, each providing a unique perspective based on his or her specialty. An effective collaborator communicates information clearly and concisely, creating a seamless transition from one provider to the next. A bad or poorly planned hand-off can result in unnecessary frustration for the medical team, increased medical costs, lengthy stays, and potential negative consequences for patients.

Interprofessional collaboration, defined as different professionals working together to achieve a common goal, is utilized in other settings besides clinical care [1]. Many research projects now integrate multiple specialties in order to incorporate findings into a larger medical picture. Education regarding the role of other disciplines is also increasingly encouraged as a way to facilitate collaboration and further knowledge.

N. Hantke, M.S. (✉)
Department of Clinical Psychology, Marquette University,
604 N. 16th Street, Milwaukee, WI, USA
e-mail: nathan.hantke@mu.edu

© Springer International Publishing Switzerland 2016
L.W. Roberts (ed.), *The Associate Professor Guidebook*,
DOI 10.1007/978-3-319-28001-1_11

Despite the often-vital role of interprofessional collaboration in medical decision-making and in research, best practice guidelines are often loosely defined. The aim of this chapter is to provide helpful advice on how to get the most out of collaborations in the three domains of research, clinical care, and education.

Research

Setting Up a Research Team

Conducting research with professionals from different fields can be stimulating and result in creative and diverse approaches. Finding and selecting research collaborators requires planning and deliberation. An experienced researcher will carefully consider all aspects of a project and the contribution each collaborator can provide. Below are examples of elements to consider when forming a collaboration:

- A collaborator should be chosen based on the needs of the project, area of expertise, and publication track record. In clinical studies, a collaborator with experience in both research and clinical care can be invaluable.
- Collaboration history, personality style, and collegiality are other attributes to consider in forming a treatment team.
- The PI should communicate clearly how emergencies should be handled, who is to be contacted, and contingency plans if that person is unavailable, particularly for research involving human subjects.

Choosing to Become a Collaborator

Being offered an opportunity to collaborate on a project can be flattering, and early-career faculty especially may readily accept without considering the situation realistically. It is easy to overextend oneself with a resulting decline in work quality and production. Before accepting a request to collaborate, consider the following:

- Is the project something that utilizes your skill set or is it a task that might be better suited to someone else?
- Is the project/research question something that interests you enough to make the time and effort expended worthwhile?
- What are the burdens and benefits to you? Will saying "yes" open professional doors? Will it help build a case for academic promotion?
- What are the reputations of the PI and other collaborators?

Make the Collaboration Work for Everyone Involved

Fostering a strong and collegial relationship can pay dividends for a researcher in the future. Not surprisingly, successful groups often continue to work together on future projects and can be highly productive. Developing this type of cohesive group has some particular challenges when collaborators are from different disciplines or have different areas of expertise. Communication becomes even more important as it is easy to assume that others have the same knowledge base and experience.

- Set clear expectations regarding roles, work division, staff supervision, data checking, and expected completion of the project.
- Discuss authorship at the onset. Most professional organizations have clear guidelines determining authorship and authorship order, but creating a consistent standard within a collaborative group can prevent future conflict.
- Be proactive in managing work with collaborators. Progress on a research project is often contingent upon feedback from collaborators. Procrastination can delay the project and be discouraging for the team.
- If your circumstances impinge on timelines, inform your colleagues. For example, professional demands may cause delays in meeting research deadlines. On the other hand, publication submission may be necessary for academic promotion or a grant submission.
- In academic centers, costs change over time (e.g., increases in annual fees, replacement of equipment, and other operating

costs). The principal investigator (PI) should draw input from collaborators to include these potential changes in a grant proposal.

- Communication by e-mail is convenient, but regularly scheduled conference calls or meetings allow interprofessional collaborators to ask questions and explain issues more fully.

- The team should set a clear itinerary for study participants based on input from involved collaborators. If a study subject has multiple stops during a day, does a research assistant meet the participant at each department? Who collects the consent form? A sloppy hand-off or disorganized agenda looks unprofessional and can deter a participant from returning.

A well-designed and organized multidisciplinary study can be productive for everyone involved. Conversely, failure to adequately plan and communicate can be frustrating and wasteful of time and resources. An interprofessional research team that is carefully selected and thoughtfully constructed can facilitate a comprehensive and integrative study.

Clinical Care

Interprofessional collaboration in clinical care has become increasingly important as research has shown that effective teamwork in a medical setting decreases medical errors and increases patient quality of care [1–3]. As a result, implementation of health care standards now explicitly requires collaboration in some instances. For example, Universal Protocol, mandated by the Joint Commission on Accreditation of Health care Organizations, requires a surgical team (including the surgeon, anesthesiologist, nurse, and surgical technician) to together perform a final time-out prior to surgery, thus reducing wrong site, wrong procedure, and wrong person surgery [4].

As health care has become increasingly competitive, a customer service model drawing on "lean" methodology used by Toyota (i.e., Toyota Production System) and other manufacturing industries is being implemented in health care settings. This patient-centered model, designed to ensure safety and quality of care by reducing inefficiency and waste, also places importance on interprofessional collaboration. For example, the interdisciplinary rounds that have been standard on inpatient acute rehabilitation units and psychiatric wards are increasingly being used on medicine units. Rounds include different specialties (e.g., pharmacy, nutrition, rehabilitation, case management, nursing, and medicine) as well as the patient and family, in some instances. These rounds, in which each patient is briefly discussed, maximize communication as the team summarizes goals, and each provider contributes to advance the plan for care and for discharge. This open communication ultimately improves patient care and decreases length of stay [5, 6].

The Institute of Medicine Committee on Quality of Health Care in America has suggested that interprofessional health care teams can best address the complex health needs of today's patients [7]. Teaching health care professionals the skills to work in a collaborative setting has becoming increasingly valued, and university health care systems have begun implementing interprofessional education programs to address this need [8].

In 2010, a joint panel of health profession schools proposed four core competencies for interprofessional collaboration in health care, which include the promotion of value and respect among professionals, being cognizant of professional roles, effective interprofessional communication, and an appreciation for the value of teamwork [9]. Unfortunately, most present-day clinicians have not received any training in interprofessional collaboration, and the following section provides some practical suggestions.

Consultation

Basic knowledge of other disciplines has been a neglected component of medical education. Even within a specialty, knowing who is best to evaluate a particular patient is often unclear. Before issuing a referral, the referring clinician may want to consider the following:

- What do I want to know? Does the referral question state my request clearly?
- Am I sending the referral to the appropriate department or person?

- If there are other referrals or tests to be performed, is there an order in which they should be done to best answer the question in a way that ensures accurate information and yet minimizes overall cost?

If unclear about the department's services or the appropriate provider, the referring clinician may consult with colleagues or a mentor, search the Internet, contact someone in the proposed department, and/or request a quick curbside consult. Requesting an in-service training may be especially helpful if it is likely there will be some overlap of care in the future.

If, on the other hand, the health care provider is serving as the consultant, he or she may find the referral question to be unclear or vague. As a consultant, you can be most effective by being proactive:

- Contact the referring provider directly via a phone call or secure e-mail to best understand what information he or she is seeking and any further history or concerns.
- Clarify who will provide feedback as this may be only one consultation in a sequence.
- Write the medical note/report clearly, minimizing jargon and avoiding acronyms and abbreviations.
- Explain how conclusions were formed and why other diagnoses may have been ruled out.
- Assume that the patient will see the report or medical note. Answer the referral question but couch it in a sensitive manner.

Coordination of Care

Communication between providers is imperative for successful clinical care. Lack of role clarification and decreased time dedicated to communication with team members can each be a factor in poor coordination of care [10]. Below are several tips for improving communication in interprofessional collaborations.

- Unless ordering a specific procedure or laboratory test, the referring provider should leave the method to answer the referral question to the consultant's expertise and discretion.

- The consultant should be sure that medical notes/reports are routed to all pertinent treating providers.

In some instances, when a patient requires specialty care on an ongoing basis, such as with a neurological illness like stroke or epilepsy, the consultant becomes a principal care provider. This new dynamic may complicate clinical care [11, 12]. Below are some tips to improve interprofessional collaboration in these situations:

- If there are multiple health care providers, the treatment team should determine who will be the point person for coordinating care.
- The report or medical note should clearly state who will follow up on suggestions and who will issue any further recommended referrals.

Education

Presenting material, whether through the larger audience of grand rounds or at a smaller departmental meeting, is an important aspect of facilitating departmental collaboration. A health care professional may be asked to perform in-service training for another department, provide his or her expertise on a difficult case, or simply present an outline of the services a specialty clinic can provide.

The purpose of the lecture will greatly influence what and how material should be covered. It is important that the lecturer is clearly informed of any expectations. For example, if the lecture is for a course, is there an expectation that the lecturer covers specific material? Should the lecture be designed to address course objectives or will there be exam questions based on the presentation? Furthermore, if the material presented is to help students prepare for a board examination, the lecturer should be notified so that he or she can adjust material accordingly.

Know the Audience

An effective presentation provides material that is at the level of the audience. This is particularly important when presenting to another discipline or several other disciplines. The presenter may want to consider the following questions when designing a presentation:

- What does my audience already know?
- If lecturing in someone else's course, what information does the professor want me to provide?

Collaborating in a Multi-Presenter Course

A course director may wish to consider using an interdisciplinary team when presenting information. This can be beneficial for several reasons. First, the inclusion of presenters from different backgrounds will likely create a well-rounded picture of the topic. Second, an interdisciplinary presentation can develop a richer understanding of how different fields interact and increase respect for the services each discipline provides. It is important, however, for the presenter to talk with his or her collaborators in advance and communicate who will cover what material.

Training Program Collaboration

In academic training programs, whether student clerkship, residency, or fellowship, all members who participate in the program must meet regularly, preferably in person to discuss the program's strengths and weaknesses. Areas of needed change can then be implemented. Setting clear expectations for program goals will reduce ambiguity.

Conclusion

One of the greatest benefits of working in an interprofessional team is the ability to utilize others' areas of expertise. For many beginning professionals, knowing who to ask and how to clearly communicate a request is sometimes more difficult than expected. The most important recommendation is to ask questions and form key contacts within your center. Taking the time to communicate clearly and frequently can be invaluable in both a research and clinical setting. Similarly, basic knowledge of other departments can facilitate effective teamwork and prevent future frustration.

Words to the Wise
- Set clear expectations regarding professional roles when collaborating on a research project. Make sure to discuss who will perform data analysis, how authorship will be determined, and who will be in charge of IRB submissions.
- When issuing a referral to another department, clearly state the question and the role of the consultant, such as who will provide feedback to the patient.
- When presenting material to other providers, take into account the knowledge base of the audience and what information is pertinent.

Ask Your Mentor or Colleagues
- Who are good resources to help you answer a question or get things done? This is important for administrative tasks as well as professional ones.
- Who has shared research interests and is a good collaborator? Is the individual's personality a good fit with yours?
- What department would be most appropriate for answering a particular clinical question? Who is a skilled professional to refer to?
- What is the culture at your center? What is the role of politics at your work?

References

1. Broers T, Poth C, Medves J. What's in a word? Understanding "interprofessional collaboration" from the student's perspective. JRIPE.
2009;1(1):3–9.
2. Campbell SM, Hann M, Hacker J, et al. Identifying predictors of high
quality care in English general practice: observational study. BMJ.
2001;323(7316):784–9.
3. Risser DT, Rice MM, Salisbury ML, Simon R, Jay GD, Berns SD. The
potential for improved teamwork to reduce medical errors in the emergency department. The MedTeams Research Consortium. Ann Emerg
Med. 1999;48(2):373–83.
4. Joint Commission on Accreditation of Health care Organizations.
Operative and post-operative complications: Lessons for the future
(Sentinel Event Alert. No.12). Oak Brook, IL; 2000.
5. Harris KT, Treanor CM, Salisbury ML. Improving patient safety with
team coordination: challenges and strategies of implementation. J Obstet
Gynecol Neonatal Nurs. 2006;35(4):557–66.
6. Curley C, McEachern JE, Speroff T. A firm trial of interdisciplinary
rounds on the inpatient medical wards: an intervention designed using
continuous quality improvement. Med Care. 1998;36(Suppl 8):AS4–12.
7. Institute of Medicine Committee on Quality of Health Care in America,
editor. Crossing the quality chasm: a new health system for the 21st century. Washington, DC: National Academy Press; 2001.
8. Bridges DR, Davidson RA, Odegard PS, Maki IV, Tomkowiak
J. Interprofessional collaboration: three best practice models of interprofessional education. Med Educ Online. 2011;16:6035.
9. Schmitt M, Blue A, Aschenbrener CA, Viggiano TR. Core competencies
for interprofessional collaborative practice: reforming health care by transforming health professionals' education. Acad Med. 2011;86(11):1351.
10. Fewster-Thuente L, Velsor-Friedrich B. Interdiscip linary collaboration
for health care professionals. Nurs Adm Q. 2008;32(1):40–8.
11. Franklin GM, Ringel SP, Jones M, Baron A. A prospective study of principal care among Colorado neurologists. Neurology. 1990;40(4):701–4.
12. Mottur-Pilson C. Primary care as form or content? Am J Med Qual.
1995;10(4):177–82.

How to Evaluate and Give Feedback

12

Jennifer R. Kogan

A key and critical component of medical education is evaluating learners and providing them with feedback. Evaluation is the process by which the academic physician assesses whether the learner has achieved the goals and objectives outlined by a course or by the clinical rotation or experience. Feedback is the impetus for improving performance. It is a fundamental cornerstone of effective teaching and learning. This chapter focuses on how to assess learners for the purpose of providing feedback. The chapter also reviews some best practices regarding the completion of evaluations.

What Is Feedback?

Feedback can be conceptualized as specific information about a learner's observed performance compared with a standard, given with the intent to improve the learner's performance. This definition highlights several important concepts. First, feedback is based

J.R. Kogan, M.D. (✉)

Department of Medicine, Perelman School of Medicine at the University of Pennsylvania, 3701 Market Street, Philadelphia, PA, USA

e-mail: Jennifer.Kogan@uphs.upenn.edu

© Springer International Publishing Switzerland 2016

155

L.W. Roberts (ed.), *The Associate Professor Guidebook*,

DOI 10.1007/978-3-319-28001-1_12

on observed performance. In the classroom setting, this could be a student's ability to apply knowledge to a problem-based learning case. In the clinical setting, feedback may focus on the core clinical skills of history taking, physical exam, interpersonal skills with patients, professionalism, and humanism. Feedback could also focus on the academic physician's observation of learners' skills related to transitions of care, interpersonal interactions with the team, oral case presentations, documentation in the medical record, or problem-solving abilities. Second, the aforementioned definition highlights that the intent of feedback is to help the learner acquire the knowledge, skills, and attitudes to improve. Third, the content of the feedback focuses on the difference in performance between how the learner is doing and a standard. For example, feedback content is about the difference between how a learner does the cardiac exam and best practices for the cardiac exam. Finally, and most important, the aim of feedback is learner improvement. Feedback is meant to be a catalyst for additional learning. It has been said that feedback is really an assessment *for* learning rather than an assessment *of* learning. In this way, the academic physician can think of himself or herself in the role of a coach for learners.

Differences Between Feedback and Evaluation

It is helpful, when thinking about feedback and evaluation, to be clear about the differences between the two. Evaluation is usually summative, meaning that it happens at the end of a defined period of time. It is about past performance, and it conveys a judgment. The purpose of evaluation is to measure a learner's achievement for the purpose of providing a grade or making decisions about progression or for certification. Evaluation is often normative (comparing one learner to other learners), but it is increasingly becoming criterion based (to what degree does the learner meet explicit standards of performance). Evaluation can be high stakes (professional certification) or low stakes (grade on quiz or assignment) or anywhere along that continuum.

In contrast, feedback is formative, meaning that it happens in real time with the intent of helping the learner develop and improve. Feedback is designed to foster learning. Feedback is about current, rather than past, performance. It is meant to convey information, reinforce strengths, and identify areas in need of improvement, "before it counts."

Types of Feedback

Feedback can further be divided into "micro-feedback" and "macro-feedback."

Micro-Feedback

Micro-, or brief, feedback is feedback in the moment. As its name suggests, it is brief, approximately 1–2 min in duration. It can be thought of as feedback nuggets. Ideally, because it is so brief, micro-feedback can, and should, be frequent (i.e., daily). An example of micro-feedback would be, "*Let me show you a better way to assess the jugular venous pressure on this patient.*" Often, this type of feedback is not recognized by the learner. Therefore, it is helpful to start micro-feedback by telling the learner that one is about to give feedback. For example, "*Let me give you some feedback about how you checked the jugular venous pressure.*"

Macro-Feedback

Macro-feedback is usually more formal. Examples of macro-feedback include sitting down with a learner after observing his or her history and physical exam or after listening to a patient or topic presentation. Macro-feedback also includes mid-rotation or mid-course feedback. Macro-feedback tends to be a sit-down conversation. It lasts longer than micro-feedback, for example 5–20 min. It tends to cover a broader array of skills and competencies. Macro-feedback tends to occur less frequently, but it is usually a more detailed conversation.

Why Is Feedback Important in Academic Medicine?

Feedback is essential in medical education so that learners can improve. To improve, learners need external information about how they are doing. This is particularly true because self-assessment, defined as an individual's assessment of personal performance or skill, is often inaccurate. Given the inaccuracy of self-assessment, self-assessment must be externally informed. This means that a learner must use not only internal data but also external data to generate an appraisal of his or her own ability.

To better understand this concept, it may be helpful to think about an analogy outside of medicine. Imagine a student who is learning to play the piano. Imagine that the student plays a piece of music. After playing, she identifies what she believes she did well and what she needs to work on. Imagine that the student never plays the piece for her teacher or someone more skilled than she. Without this external input, just how much better could the student get? How likely is it that she will be able to identify and then correct all of her mistakes?

Therefore, feedback is essential for learners. It helps learners identify their strengths and weaknesses without academic penalty. Feedback facilitates learning by providing learners with the information they need to practice and enhance their knowledge and skills. As such, feedback serves as a stimulus for professional growth. As we will see shortly, feedback should be about agreed-upon goals. Therefore, feedback clarifies the expectations of the learner.

Not only is feedback important for learners, but it is also important for teachers. Feedback done well is strongly associated with teaching ratings. Additionally, being proactive about giving feedback helps the teacher to really be cognizant of the learners' progress and their accomplishments, or lack thereof. It also provides the teacher with an opportunity to modify a course or teaching to provide more learner-centered education. That is, by understanding where the learner is, and what it is he or she needs, the teacher has an opportunity to tailor the teaching methods to the individual learners and their current abilities.

Feedback has also taken on heightened importance in this era of competency-based medical education. The focus of training and assessment is increasingly on teaching and assessing competence by documentation of achievement of the milestones. This requires ongoing assessment of trainees, with formative feedback, to ensure progression to clinical competence.

Medical Education Without Feedback

What happens when learners do not get feedback? Many problems arise. Without feedback there are missed learning opportunities. Without positive feedback, good practice is not reinforced. Without negative feedback, poor performance goes uncorrected, medical learning is incomplete, a path to improvement is not identified, and full potential may not be realized. Think back to the example of the piano student. Imagine that the student has a teacher, but the teacher only listens to the student play without ever providing any suggestions for how she might play differently. Imagine how the student's ultimate proficiency would plateau. Imagine an athlete who never is told by his coach how to get better. How good can that athlete get?

An additional problem arises when learners do not get feedback. Without feedback, learners may uphold uncorrected, inaccurate perceptions of their performance. That is, without feedback, learners may assume that they are doing a good job when, in fact, they are not. In these situations, it is not uncommon that learners will be surprised and disappointed with their final evaluations because they will think they were "doing a good job" since they received no information to the contrary. This situation can also lead to learner frustration with final evaluations because the learner, in the absence of feedback, will not feel that he or she had sufficient opportunity to improve in areas identified as needing improvement. Not uncommonly, students and residents will say that had they known there was an area of concern, they would have worked on it or changed their behaviors or attitudes. Not being given that opportunity to improve, secondary to a lack of feedback, is perceived to be unfair.

There is yet another consequence when learners do not get feedback. Without feedback, many learners will start feeling insecure about their abilities, particularly when there is no reinforcing feedback. The absence of feedback can make learners anxious and nervous because they have no sense of how they are doing and they have no idea of what they need to do to get better.

Barriers to Giving Feedback

Despite its importance, many learners are dissatisfied with the feedback that they receive, in terms of its quantity, frequency, and perceived quality. The reality is that many teachers feel uncomfortable giving feedback, and most have never had training in how to do it. In addition to a lack of training in best feedback practices, there are many additional reasons that high-quality feedback does not happen. Lack of time is frequently identified as one of the biggest barriers to giving feedback. Faculty may feel that there is inadequate time to give feedback when there are competing expectations for clinical productivity, research, scholarship, and administrative functions. In the past decade, the length of time that a teacher works with a learner, particularly in the clinical setting, has been markedly abbreviated (i.e., 1- or 2-week attending rotations). The absence of longer, more longitudinal interactions with a learner can effect feedback in multiple ways. First, faculty may feel like they have insufficient information about a learner's performance to provide feedback. Second, lack of an established learner/faculty relationship can leave faculty more uncomfortable giving feedback because they are less familiar with how a particular learner might best respond to feedback.

A very real barrier to giving feedback is providing negative feedback. Even when given constructively, there are many reasons why giving negative feedback is hard. Teachers are often concerned about undesirable consequences for the learner, such as undermining the learner's self-esteem. Faculty may worry that giving negative feedback will jeopardize the relationship they have with the trainee. Giving negative feedback may feel like giving bad news, and one may be overly negative or critical communicating this information.

What also makes feedback challenging is that it often must be delivered within the context of a flawed learner self-assessment. Feedback never occurs in a vacuum. It is given in the context of a learner's own impressions of his or her ability. The perceived value of feedback depends on the ease to which it is reconciled with the learner's self-assessment.

In addition to negative consequences for the learner, many faculty may also worry about the undesirable consequences of giving negative feedback for them as a teacher. For example, faculty may worry that giving negative feedback to a learner will reflect poorly on them as a teacher. They may be concerned that the learner will, in turn, evaluate them poorly. Faculty may then worry about the effect of these evaluations on their own advancement and promotion. Feedback:barriers

Characteristics of Effective Feedback

Knowing how to give feedback well is important to maximally help the learner. Again, feedback given well is a key catalyst to learning. Additionally, it is important to give feedback well, since feedback also has the potential to harm. For example, negative feedback, if not given correctly, can demotivate learners and actually lead to deterioration in their performance. What follows, then, are some essential characteristics of effective feedback. These characteristics, along with examples, are summarized in Table 12.1.

- *Give feedback frequently.* Think of feedback as a normal daily component of any teacher–student interaction. Up front, let the learner know that you give feedback often. You can even let your learners know early on that "no one is perfect" and "mistakes are expected" and that "everyone is here to learn." This helps to establish the expectation of daily, frequent feedback and can promote a culture that feedback is for the sake of learning. Your frequent, daily feedback or feedback nuggets (i.e., micro-feedback) then sets the stage for more comprehensive, macro-feedback later.
- *Focus feedback on agreed-upon goals.* As a teacher it is always important to set goals for your learners. You can create goals

about your course, lecture, or rotation. You can set learning goals for the week, a given day, or even a specific patient encounter. The best goals are those that are specific, clear, and concise. In addition to articulating your goals, you also should have your learners identify their learning goals too. Getting your learners to set goals is essential so that they then become active participants in the learning process by reflecting on their learning needs. In fact, the ability to frequently ask the learner what he or she desires from a teaching interaction and working with the learner to establish mutually agreed-upon goals and objectives has been associated with a proficiency in feedback skills. Once you and the learner have identified learning goals, prioritize them. Sometimes you will need to negotiate which goals to focus on. Again, the purpose of identifying goals is that this becomes the platform upon which your feedback is based. By establishing the goals, you know what to focus your observations on. Your learners will also be clear about the criteria against which their performance will be assessed. As such, it is beneficial, up front, to make sure that your learner shares with you an understanding of what your conception of good performance looks like.

- *Make feedback timely.* Feedback is best when given close to the observed activity. However, there are exceptions to this rule. Feedback given to a sleep-deprived trainee is often met with an emotional response (crying). Learners who are fatigued cannot rationally process and integrate constructive feedback. In these situations, it is often best to delay the feedback. Similarly, it is often necessary to delay feedback after a medical error because overwhelming emotions (both yours and the learners) can make it hard to both give and receive feedback.
- *Give feedback in a quiet place.* Feedback should ideally be given in a quiet, private location. This is particularly important for macro-feedback. Micro- or brief feedback is often given in the moment.
- *Signpost your feedback.* Feedback is often not recognized by learners as feedback. Therefore, it is helpful to signpost your feedback so that the learner knows it is coming and will be more likely to recognize it.

Table 12.1 Characteristics of effective feedback and examples

Feedback characteristic	Examples
Establish the expectation of frequent feedback	*"This week, I hope to give you a lot of feedback so that I can really help you to be the best doctor you can be."*
Make feedback about specific goals, both yours and the learners	*"This week, I would like for you to focus on making your patient presentations more hypothesis driven."*
	"What do you hope to get out of this course or rotation?"
	"What skills do you want to focus on this week?"
Make feedback timely	
Signpost your feedback	*"I am going to give you a little feedback now."*
	"I want to give you a little feedback on …"
	"Let me give you some feedback about …"
Start with the learner's self-assessment	*"How do you think that went?"*
	"How do you think things are going?"
	"What are you trying to work on?"
	"What do you want feedback about?"
Be specific	*"You paused often when delivering the bad news and you responded to the patient's emotion. That was really well done."* NOT *"You did a great job delivering the news."*
	"Your problem list was missing important alternative diagnoses" NOT
	"Your write-up was inadequate."
Provide positive feedback	*"Your decision to assess the patient's gait was very important for understanding potential causes for falls."*
Provide constructive feedback about areas requiring improvement	*"The history would have been more organized if you had set an agenda with the patient prior to exploring her chief complaint."*

Table 12.1 (continued)

Feedback characteristic	Examples
Prioritize feedback	
Make feedback descriptive, not evaluative	*"I thought you could have demonstrated more empathy by pausing more to listen to the patient"* NOT *"You are un-empathic and cold-hearted"*
	"I thought that a key part of the history, his occupational exposure, was omitted" NOT *"Your history was totally inadequate."*
Discuss a specific action plan	*"Focus your reading on how to distinguish systolic from diastolic murmurs"* NOT *"Read more"*
	"Practice your presentations out loud at least twice before presenting to the attending" NOT *"Work on your presentations."*

- *Start by asking for your learner's self-assessment.* There are many reasons why asking the learner for his or her own assessment is essential. First, it makes feedback an interactive conversation rather than a one-way transfer of information. Second, it helps you to assess the learner's level of insight. A self-assessment that is very different from your impression of performance is important to recognize in advance of giving feedback. Imagine giving feedback when the learner thinks his or her performance was outstanding at the same time that you believe there are significant deficiencies. That conversation will be very different from one in which the learner accurately recognizes areas of difficulty. By asking the learner to self-assess, you are also helping the learner to become better at reflection, an important skill in lifelong learning and the self-regulated profession of medicine.
- *Be specific.* Feedback should be detailed and specific. It is less helpful to provide generalities of performance (i.e., *"You did a great job."*). Although telling someone he or she did a great job makes the learner feel good, it will not help the learner advance his or her knowledge, skills, and attitudes. Feedback must describe specific behaviors.

- *Reinforce the positives*. It is important to reinforce what learners are doing well. This is more than an exercise in making the learner feel good or offering generic praise. Positive feedback should reinforce the knowledge, attitudes, or skills that you want the learner to continue to demonstrate. Ideally, focus this positive feedback on unique positive attributes of the learner, areas in which performance exceeds peers, or strengths observed during challenging or difficult circumstances (i.e., a difficult topic or a challenging clinical encounter).

- *Constructively give feedback about areas requiring improvement*. If learners are to advance in their knowledge, skills, and attitudes and improve their competence or expertise in a given domain, they need to know what requires improvement. They need to know what needs work and what they need to do better on the next time.

- *Focus feedback on directly observable behaviors*. Learners may discount feedback if they believe that the teacher does not have an accurate knowledge of their performance. Particularly as it relates to clinical skills, there is evidence that medical students and residents are observed relatively infrequently while performing many key clinical activities. Therefore, if you want to provide feedback about core clinical skills such as information gathering (history taking and physical exam), information transfer (counseling and communication of a plan), and interpersonal skills with patients and with the team, you must identify ways to be present during those activities (i.e., watching your learner with a patient; watching your learner with the team). The more you observe patient-related activities, the more likely the trainee will view you as having accurate knowledge of his or her performance. This is important to increase the learner's receptiveness to feedback.

- *Prioritize your feedback*. If you offer too much feedback at a single time, it will be difficult for the learner to process it all. If feedback is not processed, it cannot be integrated and used. Too much feedback at one time can leave the learner feeling overwhelmed and even demoralized. Therefore, you need to make decisions about how you will prioritize the feedback you want to give. Limit your constructive feedback to no more than 2–3 elements.

- *Make feedback descriptive not evaluative.* The purpose of feedback is to improve a learner's competence, not to intentionally make the learner feel bad. Therefore, you need to keep the feedback about the performance not the person. Phrasing feedback nonjudgmentally is more likely to make the feedback more acceptable and palatable to the trainee. Using the word "I" instead of "you" reinforces that what you say is your perception and can make feedback sound less accusatory.
- *Include an action plan.* Feedback without specific suggestions for how the learner can narrow the gap between current and expected or desired performance falls short in effectiveness. All feedback should have an action plan. An action plan includes the specific recommendations for how the learner will get from point A to point B. It provides information for how the learner can narrow the aforementioned gap so that he or she can advance. Action plans can be thought of as an intervention. It should provide helpful suggestions for what should the learner needs to do to acquire needed skills. As with feedback, action plans are best when they are detailed and specific.
- *Follow-up with the learner.* Because the goal of feedback is to help the learner improve, whenever possible, you should try to observe the learner again to see if your feedback was incorporated. Even if you do not have an opportunity to work with the learner again, it is still important to give feedback. In situations where you will not work with the learner again, think about how you could encourage the trainee to seek additional feedback about the identified skill area with his or her next supervisor.
- *Create a climate of trust and comfort for the learner.* You need to be giving feedback in the context of wanting to help the learner. Credible feedback is based on the perception of genuine concern for the learner and a relationship of mutual respect. Part of giving feedback is also checking your own intentions before giving feedback. Sometimes you may feel angry or upset with the learner. These feelings need to be in-check before you give feedback, because feedback really needs to come from a place of wanting to help the trainee improve.

Creating a climate of trust and comfort also means paying attention to the learner's emotional response to feedback. When you perceive such a response, you need to be ready to discuss it.

Another strategy for creating a climate of trust is to make feedback bidirectional. Learners are more likely to appreciate feedback if you also indicate early on that you welcome, expect, and also want feedback from the learner.

Approaches to Giving Feedback

It is important to know that simple do and do not rules for giving feedback underestimate the complexity inherent in how feedback should be delivered. The effectiveness of any feedback approach depends extensively on the context in which the feedback is being delivered and received. Therefore, as you think about how you want to give feedback, you need to recognize that you will need to have an inherent flexibility in your feedback approach that is based on the learner, the content of the feedback, and the context in which you are giving it.

The Feedback Sandwich

One of the most common approaches for giving feedback that people talk about is the "feedback sandwich." The feedback sandwich involves giving positive feedback first so that the trainee is receptive to what comes next. Next comes the negative feedback, the "meat of the sandwich." This is followed by additional positive feedback. Although easy to remember, there are some limitations to this approach. First, sandwiching the negative feedback may be more about the preservation of learner self-esteem. Second, the feedback sandwich quickly becomes predictable for the learner who hears the positive and then is waiting for the "but." Third, the "but" between the positive and constructive feedback often leads the learner to discount the positive feedback. And finally, this approach fails to promote a dialogue or conversation about performance since the teacher is doing all of the talking. It does not remind the teacher to get a self-assessment or end feedback with an action plan.

A Six-Step Approach

Feedback probably works best when it is a conversation between you and the learner, rather than a one-directional flow of information from you to the learner. The following six-step approach helps promote a "feedback conversation." This approach emphasizes seeking and responding to the learner's self-assessment and identifying an action plan which catalyzes future learning. It requires you to be an active listener who can reflect back what you hear. The six-step approach, along with examples, is summarized in Fig. 12.1.

Step 1. Get the learner's self-assessment about what was good about his or her performance.

Step 2. Respond to the self-assessment by identifying the strengths you agree with and any other strengths about which you want to elaborate.

Step 3. Get the learner's self-assessment about what could have been improved. This step and the next are truly the heart of the

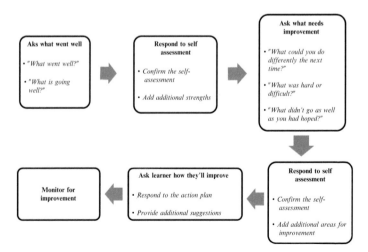

Fig. 12.1 A six-step approach to giving feedback

feedback conversation. It is these two steps where a significant proportion of the feedback time should be spent.

Step 4. Respond to the learner's self-assessment about what needed improvement. Identify what you agree with and review additional areas needing improvement.

Step 5. Ask the learner to reflect on what they might do to improve. Ask them to identify an action plan. Elaborate on the learner's response, correct it, and add to it as needed. It is very important at this point to make sure that your learner understands what he or she needs to work on and how he or she will do so.

Step 6. Monitor for improvement. Make a commitment to monitoring for improvement together. If you will not have an opportunity to work with the learner again, help the learner to identify ways to find out if he or she has successfully improved.

Difficult Feedback Situations

There are certain situations in which feedback is particularly difficult to give. Examples include giving feedback to a learner who has poor interpersonal skills or has issues with professionalism, giving feedback to the learner who really lacks insight into his or her performance, or giving feedback to the learner who is not receptive to feedback. Often, these situations involve learners who will require remediation, and this is when the academic physician will want to involve the appropriate individuals in the medical school or the course, clerkship, residency, or fellowship directors.

Feedback About Professionalism and Interpersonal Skills

Many faculty find it particularly difficult to give feedback about deficiencies in a learner's professionalism or interpersonal skills because it often feels as though that feedback is about the learner's character or personality. It may feel more subjective and also more resistant to remediation. Nevertheless, addressing lapses in professionalism or interpersonal skills is just as important as addressing a deficient fund of knowledge.

The principles of effective feedback that have been previously described still apply. When giving feedback about professionalism or interpersonal skills, it is especially important to begin by seeking out the learner's self-assessment. For example, when there are concerns about communication skills one might ask, *"How do you feel like you have been interacting with the team?"* or *"How have your interactions with your patients been?"* As with all feedback, it is especially important to be descriptive, not evaluative, describing behaviors, not the person. Using "I" statements instead of "you" statements will also make the feedback less accusatory. When providing feedback about these competencies, it can be helpful to start by saying *"The perception is that …."* For example, one might say, *"The perception is that you have seemed very short with the nurses."* Phrasing feedback this way can make its delivery easier because the learner cannot argue with a perception.

Feedback to the Learner Who Lacks Insight or Is Not Receptive

It is very challenging to give feedback to a learner who is unaware of his or her limitations or weaknesses (i.e., unconscious incompetence). The learner who lacks insight may be resistant to discussing the problem at hand, may not accept ownership or responsibility for his or her weaknesses, and may find excuses for his or her actions by blaming others or the system. Such a learner will often rationalize and/or externalize negative outcomes and therefore be resistant to getting feedback.

When giving feedback to a learner who lacks insight, try to focus the conversation on further elaborating the problem. Try to encourage additional self-assessment from the learner. Rereview expectations and try to address denial through education. The goal is to try to get the learner to identify the discrepancy between his or her present performance and the expectations or the professional standard.

Although it is difficult to receive negative feedback, most learners will be receptive because they wish to improve. However, some learners are simply not receptive to feedback. Lack of receptivity may be detected through verbal and nonverbal cues from the learner. When a learner is not receptive to feedback, it is incumbent on the academic physician to figure out why. Again, this is when one should be contacting the course director, school administration, or the training director (e.g., fellowship or program director). There is often a reason for a learner's lack of receptivity to feedback, which can be remembered by the four Ds: distraction, drugs, depression, and diagnosis. Sometimes learners are not receptive because they are distracted by issues outside of work, such as problems in a relationship, ill family members, or financial stressors. An underlying problem with substance abuse should be considered, particularly when a learner is erratic in behavior or does not seem to change behavior when expectations are explicitly set. A depressed learner also will have difficulty integrating feedback, as will a learner with any other type of personality disorder or psychiatric or medical diagnosis.

A Few Tips About Evaluation

As described earlier, evaluation is a summative assessment that occurs at the end of the time one is working with the learner. It summarizes whether the learner achieved predetermined goals and expectations. Learners can be evaluated in many ways, such as written examinations, oral exams, clinical skills exams, and 360-degrees evaluations. The most common type of assessment the academic physician will likely be asked to complete is an end-of-course, end-of-clerkship, or end-of-rotation evaluation of the learner. The criteria for assessment and the structure of the assessment form will differ from institution to institution and may also vary within the institution. What follows, therefore, are some general recommendations about how to approach completing these evaluations.

- *Familiarize yourself with the assessment form before working with the learner.* It is very important that you know what the assessment form looks like before you work with the learner. Reviewing the evaluation form tells you what competencies you will be asked to assess and will inform what types of observations you will need to make of the learner. For example, if competence in the physical exam is to be evaluated, it is incumbent upon you to figure out how to observe the learner doing a physical exam. You also must observe the learner's physical exam several times to ensure that your evaluation is reliable. Nothing frustrates a learner more than reading an evaluation when the teacher or supervisor has not directly observed the item to be assessed.

- *Do not evaluate items you have not had the opportunity to observe.* Most evaluation forms have an option for "Not applicable" or "Not observed." Use it when appropriate. Not doing so will undermine the rest of the evaluation.
- *Only write what you have reviewed during feedback.* In almost all circumstances, the learner should not read something for the first time in an evaluation. As described previously, learners will become angry to see something in their evaluation that was not communicated to them during the time you worked with them. They will feel frustrated that they were not given the opportunity to work on the area needing improvement. It is unwise to evaluate someone in an area about which he or she was not even aware that he or she was doing poorly.
- *If there is a rating scale, use the anchors.* There is tremendous grade inflation in medical education, and many evaluators restrict their ratings to the highest number on the scale. If behavioral anchors are present (i.e., examples of what a number means) read the anchors and use them when making ratings. Think critically about each item you are asked to evaluate, and try to differentiate performance in each of the different competencies. Try to rate each individual or particular skill rather than circling the same rating across all competencies.
- *If there is space for open-ended comments, make them specific.* Many assessment forms include spaces for open-ended comments. Useful comments are those that are specific, that describe relevant competencies and highlight strengths and weaknesses, providing specific examples of both. You need to know what competencies the course director is interested in so that your comments address relevant and important areas. Again, knowledge of the performance standard is needed for comments to be most

useful, because comments can than identify objectively where the trainee is compared with the expectation of where he or she should be.

- *Complete your evaluations in a timely manner.* There are several reasons why timely completion of evaluations is important. First, it can be difficult to provide a specific evaluation if months lapse between when you worked with a learner and when you complete the evaluation. Second, learners might contest the accuracy of your evaluation if it is completed months after a course or a rotation. Third, accrediting bodies (i.e., the LCME) often set standards for when students must receive evaluations or course grades. Waiting too long to complete evaluations could therefore jeopardize the school's accreditation status.

Words to the Wise
- Set goals and objectives with your learner. This is the foundation of feedback. Think of it as "feed-up." Where is the learner going?
- Increase the amount of direct observation that you do, because this is the focus of your feedback. Talk with a colleague about feasible strategies for increasing the amount of direct observation you do.
- Seek the learner's self-assessment before you give feedback. Really listen and respond to what the learner has to say.
- Include positive (reinforcing) and negative (constructive) feedback that is specific, objective, timely, and prioritized. It should answer the question, "What progress is being made toward the goal?"
- Make sure that your feedback has an action plan. Your feedback should "feed-forward" and answer the question "What activities need to be undertaken to make progress?" or "Where to next?"
- Role-play with a mentor or a colleague to practice difficult feedback.
- Consider participating in a workshop about teaching skills or providing feedback to practice your skills.

Ask Your Mentor or Colleagues
- What types of feedback have been challenging for you to give? What made them challenging?
- What strategies have you used to give challenging feedback?
- Was there a time you did not give a trainee feedback and wish you had? Why do you think that happened? How could you prevent it from happening again?

Further Reading

Archer JC. State of the science in health professional education: effective feedback. Med Educ. 2010;44: 101–8.

Branch Jr WT, Paranjape A. Feedback and reflection: teaching methods for clinical settings. Acad Med. 2002;77:1185–8.

Cantillon P, Sargeant J. Giving feedback in clinical settings. BMJ. 2008; 337:1292–4.

Ende J. Feedback in clinical medical education. JAMA. 1983;250:777–81.

Hattie J, Timperley H. The power of feedback. Rev Educ Res. 2007; 77:81–112.

Mann K, van der Vleuten C, Eva K, et al. Tensions in informed self-assessment: how the desire for feedback and reticence to collect and use it can conflict. Acad Med. 2011;86:1120–7.

Mazor KM, Holtman MC, Shchukin Y, Mee J, Katsufrakis PJ. The relationship between direct observation, knowledge, and feedback: results of a national survey. Acad Med. 2011;86(10):S63–8.

Menachery EP, Knight AM, Kolodner K, Wright SM. Physician characteristics associated with proficiency in feedback skills. J Gen Intern Med. 2006;21:440–6.

Milan FB, Parish SJ, Reichgott MJ. A model for educational feedback based on clinical communication skills strategies: beyond the "feedback sandwich". Teach Learn Med. 2006;18(1):42–7.

Van de Ridder JMM, Stokking KM, McGaghie WC, ten Cate OTJ. What is feedback in clinical education? Med Educ. 2008;42:189–97.

How to Be a Good Mentor

13

Jonathan F. Borus

Most academic physicians and scientists already have "full plates" of clinical, teaching, research, and administrative responsibilities. However, mentoring is a vital role in which faculty members provide an invaluable service to our "young" by devoting the time and energy necessary to mentor them to be successful during their training years and careers. Trainees and early-career faculty often are new to the city, institution, department, and/or laboratory in which they are working and need to learn both "how it is done here" and how things are done in the field in general. Mentees are especially needy of wise and experienced counsel about how to get the most out of their institution and its people and resources. Even though there is usually no immediate quid pro quo for mentoring, and often it is not a well-paid or academically rewarded role, if we do not take on this essential faculty role we are neglecting our duty to both the next generation and the future of our field.

J.F. Borus, M.D. (✉)
Department of Psychiatry, Brigham and Women's Hospital
and Harvard Medical School, 75 Francis Street, Boston, MA, USA
e-mail: jborus@partners.org

© Springer International Publishing Switzerland 2016   175
L.W. Roberts (ed.), *The Associate Professor Guidebook*,
DOI 10.1007/978-3-319-28001-1_13

Should/Can All Faculty Members Be Mentors?

All successful mentors must be generative, willing to give of themselves to be helpful to their mentee, able to listen to their mentees' issues and perspectives rather than impose their own, and willing to put their mentees' needs ahead of their own. It is an unfortunate reality that some faculty members do not inherently possess these generative, non-narcissistic qualities; such faculty members often fail as mentors and therefore probably should not be assigned to this role in the first place. The inability to take the mentee's perspective and focus primarily on the mentee's skill and career development can make a mentor unhelpful and often harmful to a mentee.

A mentor can be unhelpful to his or her mentee in many ways. Examples include the mentor who wants the mentee to only work on the mentor's personal research, even though this is not the primary area the mentee wants to pursue; the mentor who wants the mentee to become a clone, a "mini me," and does not provide sufficient space for the mentee to explore and become what he or she wants to be or might be best at; the mentor who cannot "let go" of the mentee and insists that the latter, and at times former mentees, continues to work in the mentor's area and/or publish with the mentor when the mentees need to demonstrate independence to advance their careers; the mentor who does not support or tries to block a mentee from leaving his or her current role or institution to work elsewhere; and the mentor who does not provide sufficient time for the mentoring relationship or adequate encouragement for the mentee, therefore inhibiting the mentee's development. Unfortunately, some of us have experienced the detrimental effects of such mentors, and we must maintain constant self-awareness about these possible issues in our own mentoring relationships.

Types of Mentors

There are two basic types of mentors, technical mentors and developmental mentors, with each type providing different things to its mentees.

A *technical mentor* is a more-senior practitioner who is expert in a particular area, skill, or task that the more-junior mentee wants or needs to master. The technical mentor's role is to teach, supervise, guide, and advise the mentee about that area, skill, or task to help the latter achieve competence in it, and the mentee often works with or under the mentor. The technical mentor, therefore, may be the mentee's "boss," with responsibility for evaluating the mentee's work and productivity in that area, skill, or task.

In contrast, a *developmental mentor* is a more-senior practitioner of the general area or field in which the mentee needs to learn or work but need not necessarily be an expert in the exact area or perform the specific task or skill the mentee wants to master. The developmental mentor's role is to advise the mentee about more general institutional and career issues, help the mentee think through his or her career development possibilities, and link the mentee with others both within and external to their common organization who might further the mentee's career, including technical mentors who can help the mentee master specific skills. In contrast to the technical mentor, the developmental mentor usually has no responsibility for the mentee's work, productivity, or evaluation.

An important difference between technical and developmental mentors is the former's evaluative role. This role introduces an inherent conflict of interest into the relationship for both mentor and mentee. It may inhibit mentees' open discussion of professional priorities or career possibilities that differ from those of their technical mentor and make it more difficult for the mentor to openly support a broad exploration of possibilities that might lead to a change in the current work being done within the scope of the mentor's responsibility. The mentor with responsibility for evaluating his or her mentee's work product may find it more difficult to provide counsel and advice that meets the mentee's general career needs if these veer from the primary goal of achieving expertise and productivity in the technical mentor's field. For example, a mentee who does research in his or her mentor's lab will find it difficult to discuss moving to another lab or into a different area of investigation that might limit work on the technical mentor's project. In contrast, the developmental mentor, who does not have such evaluative responsibility, will not have a conflict about discussing a range of possibilities for his or her mentee's professional development.

Although mentees need both types of mentors to be successful, and the roles do have some overlap, most faculty members are better at one type than the other. On occasion, the same person can be both the developmental and technical mentor of a particular mentee, but it is a difficult tightrope to walk. For example, over the years I was the Department Chair, I had many mentees, some of whom were faculty in my department. I was aware of the inherent role conflict when faculty mentees would come to talk about changes in their priorities and potential job opportunities elsewhere if I wanted ("needed") them to continue to fill specific roles in my department. I would acknowledge this conflict to such mentees and say that although as Chair I wanted them to stay in the department, I would do my best to "take off my Chair hat" to help explore their full range of professional possibilities and what was currently best for their career and personal situation. However, it is important to help our mentees understand that no one person can or will meet all of their mentoring needs. Both trainees and faculty thrive if they can develop a network of mentors, multiple helpful people who can provide mentoring about different aspects of academic life.

Initiating and Structuring the Mentoring Relationship

Mentoring relationships are initiated in two main ways. Some departments suggest that their trainees and new faculty members become familiar with the department on their own and invite them to ask more-senior faculty members to be their mentors. Other departments assign new arrivals to either or both technical and developmental mentors with the understanding that the pair will try out this relationship to see if it is helpful to the mentee and, if it does not work for either party, there can be a "no fault" termination of the relationship. The advantage of making an initial mentor assignment to new trainees or faculty members, rather than letting them scramble to find their own mentors, is that it links mentees early on with faculty knowledgeable about the department who can guide the mentee to needed organizational resources. If this initial pairing is not a good fit, the first mentor can help steer the mentee toward a more appropriate ongoing mentor. However, whether by invitation or department assignment, mentors should not accept new mentees if they do not have adequate time, professional "space" and energy, or the desire to be a mentor, as without these, the relationship will not benefit either party. If such mentoring is primarily an unrecognized "add-on" to a faculty member's already full plate of duties and unrewarded with money, academic credit, and/or time, it is unlikely to be successful.

It is the mentor's role to structure the relationship with the mentee. At the outset, mentors and mentees should explore and define the goals of their relationship to facilitate agreement on how to best operate to achieve them. Successful mentoring relationships require agreed-upon boundaries, roles, and responsibilities, and both mentor and mentee must devote sufficient time and energy to this relationship with clear, agreed-upon expectations of how it will work. The mentor should outline the frequency and length of meetings, expectations of inter-meeting work by each party, and an initial time frame for the relationship. The latter is necessary to set the expectation that the relationship will be periodically evaluated by both parties to be sure that it is helpful to the mentee and not overly onerous on the mentor.

This structure may be written up in a formal "mentoring contract," but even without a contract it is important that the expectations of both parties are clear, understood, and agreed to early in the relationship. Without such an agreement, informal advising and other senior faculty/trainee or junior faculty interactions can be misinterpreted as a mentoring relationship with negative consequences. Although informal "hit-and-run" advice and curbside counseling can be helpful, they may mistakenly encourage the junior person to believe that a senior person is his or her mentor when the latter has not made such a commitment, which can lead to expectations not being met and a lack of needed mentoring.

Difficult Mentoring Relationships for the Mentor

At times, mentees have unrealistic expectations of their mentors. Examples include the relatively new mentee who expects the technical mentor to affirm competence that the mentee has not yet demonstrated, the mentee who expects the mentor to provide recommendations and entrée to colleagues and organizations which the mentee has not yet earned, and the mentee who does not fulfill his or her responsibilities to the mentoring relationship, such as coming unprepared to mentoring meetings, not doing the agreed-upon interim work, and otherwise being "wasteful" of the mentor's time and expertise. At other times, the mentee's skills may be beyond those of the mentor, and the mentor is unwilling to acknowledge this reality and then help the mentee find a more appropriate mentor. It is important that mentors provide direct feedback to their mentees (and vice versa) about how the relationship is going and that there be periodic, bidirectional evaluation of the mentoring relationship to be sure that it is meeting the needs and expectations of both parties. A mentoring relationship that does not work after a reasonable trial period and appropriate feedback should be terminated. It is hoped that this will be a rare occurrence accompanied by an explanation of the reasons the mentor or mentee feels the relationship is not working and, if possible, by referral of the mentee to another potential mentor. With academic time and energy always scarce resources, an unhelpful, nonproductive mentoring relationship should not be allowed by either party to drift along ad infinitum.

Mentoring Across Differences

Mentoring relationships by definition involve two people at different points in the academic hierarchy who come to the relationship with differing levels of knowledge, expertise, and experience. In addition, other differences between mentor and mentee should be acknowledged if the relationship is to be successful and ultimately most helpful to the mentee. These include mentoring relationships in which the mentor and mentee are of different genders, races, and/or generations. In such "cross-identity" mentoring relationships, the mentor has the obligation early on to begin a discussion of the differences between himself or herself and the mentee, expressing eagerness to learn about the mentee's background, views, and understanding of the relationship and the field. Such an invitation by the mentor will make it easier for the mentee to be open about these differences and promote more shared understanding of often differing views of the situation/

institution in which they are working. Even when mentor and mentee are of the same gender, race, and generation, discussion of "where they are coming from" near the beginning of the mentoring relationship will reveal other differences in their backgrounds and personal and professional priorities that are best acknowledged so that they add to, rather than inhibit, the mentoring relationship.

Developing Your Mentoring Abilities

Mentors are *both* born and made. For faculty members who do possess the inherent generativity necessary for the mentoring role, there are ways to learn how to improve their abilities to be more helpful to mentees. We would not think of sending faculty members to treat patients, undertake research, or teach without training and supervision until they can demonstrate basic levels of competence in these roles. Just because faculty members have been someone else's mentee at some point during their careers does not mean that they are knowledgeable about mentoring or could not do it better with training, supervision, and consultation. Too frequently we send faculty to be mentors of early-career colleagues without such preparation and then leave them isolated in this role, often leading to mentors becoming frustrated at their inability to be helpful to their mentees and giving up on this role. Mentors need opportunities to learn more about the mentoring role and discuss their mentoring experiences. These can include obtaining supervision on mentoring; seeking consultation about difficult mentoring situations or issues; accessing "mentoring toolkits" and other resources that provide references, best practice models, and other tools to use in mentoring; and taking formal mentoring courses (such as the one described in the subsequent text). All mentors need to have mentoring supervision and/or consultation readily available and then must be encouraged to use such help when they face difficult or complex mentoring issues.

At Brigham and Women's Hospital in Boston over the past 4 years, we have offered a course to help established faculty mentors improve their mentoring skills. The "Faculty Mentoring Leadership Program" (FMLP) was stimulated by a 2008 all-faculty survey, which found that junior faculty wanted more mentoring and experienced faculty who already were providing such mentoring wanted to learn how to be better mentors. To date, FMLP has trained three cohorts of faculty members (68 in total) from most of the hospital's departments with the goals of enhancing their mentoring skills and leadership and creating a supportive community of mentors across the hospital. As a prerequisite for acceptance into FMLP, faculty members must have at least 5 years' experience mentoring other faculty to demonstrate their investment in this role and be willing to commit to attending all of the program's 9 monthly meetings. Each of these meetings focuses on specific mentoring issues, including the benefits of mentorship; what is and is not mentoring; structuring the mentoring relationship's expectations and boundaries; difficult and/or complex mentoring situations; mentoring across generational, gender, and racial differences; mentoring networks; the life course of mentorship; mentoring and the mentor's career; and feedback within the mentoring relationship. We have found that the most effective way to approach each of these issues is through interactive case-based discussions, with the case materials derived directly from the participants' experiences as mentors and mentees and then woven into anonymous representative cases that focus on the session's topic. Evaluation of FMLP's first (2009–2010) cohort, immediately after the course and at 6-month follow-up, found significant improvements in the participants' self-reported mentoring effectiveness and ability to accomplish their mentoring goals, as well as a positive effect on their careers.

The Life Course of Mentorship

As mentioned previously, all mentoring relationships should begin with a structure that includes an expected initial length with renewal possible by mutual agreement. But how long should a mentoring relationship continue? Mentors:and menteesMentors:and menteesMentors:and menteesboth the mentor and the mentee make it impractical to continue. If either leaves the institution, a previously successful mentoring relationship can be continued long distance via phone or e-mail. The problem with continuing long distance as the primary mentoring relationship is the difficulty the mentor often has maintaining commitment to a mentee at another institution; once the mentor assumes new activities and responsibilities, including working with new local mentees, providing sufficient time and energy for a former mentee becomes difficult. In such circumstances, it is best for the mentor to help the mentee find a new primary mentor at the mentee's institution, with continued long-distance mentoring becoming an auxiliary part of the mentee's larger mentoring network.

At some point, mentors need to "let go" and allow their mentees to gain the independence necessary for career advancement and academic promotion. Some technical mentors in particular have difficulty giving up control of their mentees' careers and authorship on their mentees' papers, even though this is not in their mentees' best interest. As mentioned earlier, at any time when it is clear to the mentor or mentee that the relationship is no longer productive or helpful, after appropriate feedback and discussion the relationship should be terminated.

Most mentoring relationships do end, and academic faculty members usually have several different mentors over the course of their careers related to the faculty member's stage of professional development, institution, and professional focus. Former mentors often continue to play important ancillary roles, and their mentees may call upon them to discuss complex issues. In such cases, however, the former mentor and his or her former mentee must be aware that distance from the intricacies of the latter's current situation may make the mentor's advice less specifically helpful than previously, or conversely, provide an objective viewpoint from which the mentor can offer impartial advice.

Rewards for Mentors

To some extent, mentoring, like virtue, is its own reward. Being helpful to the next generation is in and of itself a gratifying reward. It provides the opportunity to give back, to be altruistic, and to have a hand in nurturing and guiding the next generation. In addition, technical mentors often receive assistance from mentees who work in the mentor's area as part of the relationship, and this may help advance the mentor's productivity and career. In some academic institutions, a track record of successful mentoring, with a listing of successful mentees on the mentor's CV, has a positive influence on promotion decisions. Some institutions and departments also have formal mentoring awards, although these are relatively rare when compared to the large amount of mentoring needed in any academic setting. The major rewards for the mentor are the gratitude of his or her mentees and the good feeling the mentor gets from having helped the leaders of the next generation explore, shape, and succeed in whatever path they have chosen. One of the greatest pleasures for me in having mentored many trainees and faculty over the course of my academic career has been to have former mentees, many of whom have professional accomplishments that far surpass mine, still seek me out to talk about their lives and careers. Having helped them on their way up, I have found that, in a reversal of roles, former mentees have now been helpful to me in the later years of my professional career, which may be the ultimate reward for a lifetime of mentoring (Table 13.1).

Table 13.1 Nine characteristics of the good mentor

1. Sets clear boundaries on, and expectations for, the mentoring relationship
2. Is trustworthy and encourages the mentee to openly explore possibilities with the mentor, knowing that appropriate confidentiality will be maintained
3. Listens thoughtfully to the mentee's experience, issues, and problems
4. Explains how things "work" in their common field and institution and helps guide the mentee through the system
5. Encourages and helps the mentee explore career possibilities
6. Connects the mentee to other mentors, important people inside and outside of the institution, and organizations that might be helpful to the mentee's career
7. Runs interference and helps eliminate barriers to the mentee's professional development
8. Provides direct, nonevaluative feedback to the mentee about ways he or she could improve professionally
9. Acknowledges that mentoring is an asymmetric relationship in which the mentee's needs come first, with the primary focus always on the mentee's development, not the mentor's advancement

Words to the Wise
- Do constantly remain aware that your first mentoring obligation is to your mentee's development rather than your own career.
- Do explore how mentoring can help your career advancement and other possible rewards for mentoring.
- Do provide direct, nonevaluative feedback to your mentee when you are aware of ways the mentee could be more effective.
- Do learn more about mentoring via courses and/or supervision, and get consultation from colleagues in difficult mentoring situations.
- Do not take on a mentoring relationship in which you cannot be generative, responsible, and provide the necessary time and energy, without it causing excessive strain on your other responsibilities.
- Do not take on a mentoring relationship in which you need more from the mentee than he/she does from you.
- Do not continue a mentoring relationship that isn't working, including those in which your mentee is not fulfilling his/her responsibilities or you cannot fulfill yours.
- Do not prolong mentoring relationships if they inhibit the independence and career development of your mentee.

Ask Your Mentor or Colleagues
- Where can I get consultation about a difficult mentoring situation?
- How and where can I get help to learn how to be a better mentor?
- What should I do if my mentee wants to go in a direction in which I am not expert?
- How can being a mentor help advance my career at our institution?

Acknowledgment The author acknowledges the helpful comments of Audrey Haas, M.B.A.; Carol C. Nadelson, M.D.; Ellen W. Seely, M.D.; and Lawrence Tsen, M.D., in determining the final version of this chapter.

Further Reading

Detsy AS, Baerlocher MO. Academic mentoring—how to give it and how to get it. JAMA. 2007;297:2134–6.

Feldman MD. Mentoring facilitator tool kit, UCSF Faculty mentoring program. Regents of the University of California; 2010.

Kram KE, Higgins MC. A new approach to mentoring. MIT Sloan management review. New York: Harvard Business School Publishing; 2004.

Meister JC, Willyerd K. Mentoring millennials. Harv Bus Rev. 2010;88(5):68–72.

Sambunjak D, Marusic A. Mentoring: what's in a name? JAMA. 2010;302:2591–2.

Sambunjak D, Straus SF, Marusic A. Mentoring in academic medicine: a systemic review. JAMA. 2006;296:1103–15.

Thomas DA. Race matters: the truth about mentoring minorities. Harv Bus Rev. 2001;79:98–107.

Tsen L, Borus JF, Nadelson CC, Seely EW, Haas A, Fuhlbrigge AL. The development, implementation, and assessment of an innovative mentoring leadership program for faculty mentors. Acad Med 2012 Oct 22 [Epub ahead of print] PMID: 23095917

Worley LM, Borus JF, Hilty DM. Being a good mentor and colleague. In: Roberts LW, Hilty DM, editors. Handbook of career development in academic psychiatry and behavioral sciences. Washington, DC: American Psychiatric Publishing Inc; 2007. p. 293–8.

How to Strengthen Your Own and Others' Morale

14

Michael D. Jibson

Morale is the collective measure of job satisfaction, personal well-being, quality of interactions, and activity level of individuals that work together. This chapter addresses how to build an environment that supports and enhances the job satisfaction of the people with whom you work and for whom you are responsible. The principles presented are equally applicable to a clinical teaching service, laboratory group, residency program, department, or medical school. They are less about how to succeed in formal administrative roles and more about specific behaviors that enhance the morale of everyone you supervise, direct, or with whom you collaborate.

Despite its recognition as an essential component of a successful organization and a core responsibility of leaders, relatively little attention has been paid to the factors that drive resident and faculty morale in the medical literature [1, 2]. Extensive work within the field of organizational behavior has focused primarily on the business community [3], whose goals and methods may overlap with but are not identical to those of healthcare in general or medical education in particular. Consequently, the following are suggested best practices based on observations of groups that succeeded or failed to work well together in academic medicine.

M.D. Jibson, M.D., Ph.D. (✉)
Department of Psychiatry, University of Michigan Health System,
1500 E. Medical Center Dr., Ann Arbor, MI, USA
e-mail: mdjibson@med.umich.edu

© Springer International Publishing Switzerland 2016
L.W. Roberts (ed.), *The Associate Professor Guidebook*,
DOI 10.1007/978-3-319-28001-1_14

They begin with four basic principles that are applicable across a range of situations (Table 14.1). These will be followed by a series of specific issues that require special attention.

Table 14.1 Essential qualities to strengthen morale

For the faculty member/supervisor	For the academic administrator
Engagement	
• Accept your role as a leader	• Lead by moral (not administrative) authority
• Recognize the people who depend on you	• Be visible, involved, and active
• Respect their roles and work	• Recognize the work and achievements of individuals and groups
• Facilitate smooth working relationships	
Support	
• Be respectful and empathic	• Know your trainees, faculty, and staff
• Emphasize the positive Morale:qualities	• Facilitate personal and professional growth
• Avoid condescension and implied criticism	• Give priority to individuals' needs over administrative convenience
• Share your experience and perspectives	• Confront problems promptly and respectfully
Transparency	
• Be clear, fair, and consistent	• Build a culture of openness, fairness, and integrity
• Be specific about your expectations Morale:qualities	• Seek input and consensus whenever possible
• Give prompt, specific feedback	• Be consistent and fair in setting priorities
• Accept feedback from others	• Explain the basis for decisions and policies
Balance	
• Be clear and open about your interests and goals	• Know your trainees and faculty
• Seek areas of alignment between your interests and the needs of the department	• Be clear about the program or department's priorities
• Be responsible with the autonomy you are given Morale:qualities	• Facilitate appropriate autonomous activity
	• Say "Yes," whenever possible; say "No," whenever necessary

General Principles

Be Engaged

Leadership is fundamental to academic medicine. From the clinical instructor supervising a medical student to the dean managing a medical school, academic life inevitably includes responsibility for the welfare of the people around you. Engagement means recognition and acceptance of your responsibility as a leader. The capacity to encourage and empower your trainees and colleagues does not arise from administrative authority, but from a personal interest in them and a genuine desire to facilitate their work and professional development. Your goal should be for trainees and faculty to accept your directions not because of your position, but because they know you care about them, understand their concerns, are fair, and have good reasons for your decisions. It should never come down to them doing something because you have the power to force them. Ironically, this principle of leadership is easier to learn at the bottom of the academic ladder than at the top.

Every faculty member works within an academic and healthcare hierarchy that has expectations of performance and grants autonomy within the unavoidable limits of institutional mission, financial priorities, regulatory requirements, and administrative directives. Although it is easy to see the organizational chart extending above you (seemingly to infinity, as every chair has discovered), it is equally important even as an entry-level faculty member to recognize who is depending on you and how you can serve them.

Take a moment to notice the people who are looking to you for direction. Most conspicuous are likely to be the medical students and house officers assigned to your clinical service. Consider your role in terms of their needs. You are responsible to provide them with direction, to serve as a role model, and to create an environment that facilitates their professional growth. They will soon be your colleagues; treat them as such and help them get there.

Next you may notice allied health or technical professionals, such as nurses, social workers, laboratory technicians, activity therapists, dieticians, and innumerable others. You are responsible for their integration into clinical and research operations. Their work is essential to yours; help them do it. You will inevitably encounter clerical and administrative staff. The paperwork they handle may seem an annoyance or even a hindrance to your work, but no system can operate without them; comply with their requests and they will keep you on track and in compliance with critical regulations. Less conspicuous may be the housekeeping, maintenance, and security staff. Much of their work is invisible; that does not mean it should be overlooked. All of these workers are skilled at what they do and take their responsibilities as seriously as you do yours; respect their roles, their training, their professionalism, and their judgment. None of these people really work for you, but sometimes they may have to follow your directions (e.g., medical orders), and they are always affected by how you lead (see Case Study #1).

In the normal flow of academic life as your career progresses, formal leadership roles are expected. The skills you develop early in your career will serve you well as you take on these responsibilities. Your challenge will be to fully assume the role you are assigned and learn to adapt your relationships to the new position.

As your administrative role grows, so do your obligations to faculty, trainees, and auxiliary staff. They need to know that someone is at the helm directing everyone's efforts and protecting them from threats to their own goals, priorities, and job security. Be active and visible in the role. Few things undermine staff morale more than their feeling unnoticed and unappreciated. Give people the assurance that you are there and are aware of their work, their needs, the rules that govern them, and the forces that affect them. Regular acknowledgement of their challenges and achievements is an important element of group leadership. Invisible or absentee leadership rarely engenders confidence, enhances energy, or facilitates individual or group success. If 80 % of success is showing up, make sure you are there (see Case Study #2).

One effective approach is to be present on the front lines of the work. Administrators who sit in distant offices making decisions about work hours, clinical quotas, and staffing ratios are unlikely to fully grasp the impact of their policies on job satisfaction or the work environment. Leaders who maintain a clinic schedule, cover an inpatient service, and schedule themselves for regular call shifts gain insight and credibility available no other way.

Additional efforts may be required to identify career milestones such as awards and publications; personal events such as birthdays, births, and deaths; and individual issues such as medical or family problems. The extra effort to ask about these things periodically not only communicates interest but allows you to appreciate that you are surrounded by real, three-dimensional people. They will respond accordingly.

Be Supportive

Relationships with colleagues are an important source of job satisfaction [4, 5]. To make the most of this resource, it is essential that relationships be positive, constructive, and supportive. Support for individuals covers a broad range of intellectual, emotional, social, and academic needs experienced by trainees, faculty, and other staff. Support for these needs may be offered up or down the chain of command, laterally among peers, and elsewhere. It may take the form of personal warmth, career advice, clinical consultation, research collaborations, or any number of other means by which the interests of another person become paramount. As a general attitude, several elements are essential.

Be respectful in every interaction [6]. Recognize the worth of the person you are seeing as a professional (or potential professional), a colleague, and a fellow human being. Seek to understand his or her perspective, feelings, and needs. Ask yourself how you might be most helpful and follow through on your thoughts, if only with a word. Be aware of the unspoken implications of your feedback and recommendations regarding the value of a person's skills, interests, and potential. Few things are as demoralizing as disregard or condescension [7]; take care to emphasize the positive and to convey your respect and desire to be helpful.

Support does not always mean agreement. Confrontation of incorrect information or maladaptive responses may be the most constructive response [8]. In some cases, it may even be helpful to directly question someone's priorities or goals. Faulty understanding of the facts is relatively easy to detect and is essential to correct. Take the time to probe how your trainee or colleague understands things; be straightforward in addressing errors of fact. Errors of interpretation are equally important but may be harder to counteract. Be willing to share your perspective on what is happening behind the scenes and on the implicit meaning of policies and decisions. Care enough to confront maladaptive behaviors; do not stand by and allow a trainee to unknowingly build a reputation as oppositional, high maintenance, or entitled. Prompt, focused feedback on these behaviors is hard to give and painful to receive, but is essential to professional development. Good reality testing is a precious service, even when that reality hurts.

Be attentive to individuals' career development. Programs and departments differ in the degree to which work assignments are allocated based on the needs of the department versus the interests of the individual. The morale of trainees is closely correlated with their perception of the educational value of their clinical rotations as compared to the service needs of the department. The attachment faculty members feel to the institution will be affected by whether they perceive that their positions represent a positive career move or just fill gaps in clinical or research operations. From an administrative perspective, policies differ as to whether they primarily serve the department or its individual members. For example, when taking corrective action, a training program may have a low threshold for termination in order to maintain the integrity and reputation of the program or may favor extensive remediation in the hope that every trainee will successfully reach graduation. To some degree, the difference is how these issues are framed. More substantive is how they are actually approached. As a steward over the education of trainees and career growth of faculty, remember that their success is your success and their morale is dependent on your support (see Case Study #3).

Be Transparent

Regular, high-quality communication facilitates every aspect of clinical care, education, and administration. In contrast, job satisfaction and performance suffer when policies are announced without context, decisions are made without discussion, and evaluations are issued without prior expectations. Even controversial or difficult decisions will be accepted more readily if the process by which they are reached is explained. Similarly, summative feedback should be the culmination of a series of earlier communications about performance. The endpoints of these processes should not be their only visible feature.

Transparency promotes both the reality and the appearance of fairness and integrity. These are essential qualities of leadership that build confidence and satisfaction among trainees and faculty [9]. Openness in decision-making encourages a balanced approach and carries with it a built-in corrective for bias and favoritism. It builds trust in the leader and demonstrates the leader's trust in the group. This working relationship encourages an alignment of individuals' values and goals with those of the institution. Beware of decisions that you do not want to be widely known; this is a warning sign that your integrity is compromised. As a general rule, it is a poor policy that is based on not being exposed.

Whether as a supervisor or administrator, be clear about your expectations for trainees, faculty, and others for whom you are responsible. Establish standards of performance, explain how they will be monitored, and provide frequent feedback on how each person is doing relative to those standards and to their peers. Meet with them regularly to review expectations and performance. Be clear when standards are not being met and about the consequences of nonperformance (see Case Study #4).

As a supervisor and as an administrator, transparency works both ways. Listen to others' opinions and be open to different perspectives. Make it clear that you have heard what they have to say and that you are taking their views into account. Decisions made by consensus have a power not shared by administrative decrees, providing greater understanding and acceptance. For those issues that must be decided by a smaller group, take not one but two moments to explain your decisions: first to share the background information that informed your choice and then to review the rationale you followed. Even those who disagree will at least have the correct information in front of them and will know the basis on which the decision was made.

Balance Direction and Autonomy

Productivity and a positive work environment require a constructive interaction between the leader and members of a group [7, 10]. Professional satisfaction and effectiveness improve when the goals and methods of the group are clear to everyone and their efforts are united [11]. Leaders give direction and structure to group endeavors; workers provide the energy and productivity necessary to accomplish them. Good leaders motivate not only through support and clarity of expectation but also through clarity of vision; good workers accept that vision as their own and align their activities with it.

The directive nature of leadership stands in contrast to the need to promote independence among the members of the group. Medicine is hardly the place to find individuals who will be satisfied with subservient roles and rote activities. Little wonder, then, that personal control over job descriptions and work hours are among the most common factors cited in studies of physician morale, among both faculty and residents [12–14]. Part of the role of a faculty member is to find ways to grow professionally; part of the role of a leader is to facilitate that independent activity and growth in others.

A key challenge of life in academic medicine is to balance these seemingly incompatible goals [15]. The least elegant approach is for the administrative leader to give everyone control over a few things and to retain control over everything else. More effective strategies include the exploration of convergent interests, education and persuasion, job matching, and creative negotiation. Faculty at all levels have a role to play in this process.

Convergent interests are those areas in which what someone wants to do and what the administration needs him or her to do are the same. This is an essential element of contract negotiation for a new faculty member. To be effective, both parties need to be clear about their goals and motivations. As an entry-level faculty member, think carefully about your priorities, interests, and dislikes. Keep in mind that an activity that you found tolerable for a few months of residency may be less so when telescoped over decades. If your true motivation for taking a job is only partially related to the job description (e.g., you want to teach medical students, but the only faculty job available is on an inpatient unit you barely survived as a resident), say so before you sign the contract.

As a senior administrator in the department, be clear about the prospects of career development and flexibility of assignment for a new faculty member. The two of you must work creatively to match personal interests with departmental needs, and each must be willing to adjust expectations.

This process will go on as interests and job descriptions evolve over the course of a career. Much of your contribution to your own career development as a faculty member is your ability to find professional interests that will benefit your department. Much of your contribution to faculty as an administrator will be your ability to find the right person to meet a need in the department. The right person is not only the person with the right skills but also the right interests and career goals. If that faculty member is not obvious, opportunities for faculty training may develop both the interest and the skills the department needs.

For trainees, the process has the added dimension of certification requirements. Students and residents must achieve certain competencies to graduate, and the department has an obligation to make those available and to facilitate the process. Education directors must maintain the quality and integrity of their programs. Consequently, certain activities and standards cannot be neglected or compromised. Even with these constraints, however, it is possible to introduce a measure of independence to the process. Directors of medical student education can offer a variety of clerkship options and can direct students to the sites most compatible with their interests. Residency program directors can be flexible with scheduling, creative with electives, and active in arranging faculty mentors. A simple rule to follow when a trainee asks to deviate from the standard schedule is, "Say, 'Yes,' whenever possible; say, 'No,' whenever necessary."

Specific Issues

The general principles just described come into play in a variety of situations, a few of which are delineated below. These are specific areas that will be especially important to the morale of trainees and faculty. They are described from the perspective of the person best positioned to have an impact on the group dynamic.

Supervision and Mentorship

The learning environment is among the most important factors cited by residents in the quality of their training experiences [16], and no one has a more profound effect on that environment than the clinical supervisor. It is essential that faculty master the skills needed to oversee the work of their trainees, recognize their strengths and weaknesses, guide them toward a mastery of the field, and support them in their struggle to achieve it.

As a supervisor, be clear about your expectations and your standards. Accrediting bodies for both medical schools and residencies require that every training experience has explicit learning objectives and that these be made clear from the outset to the trainee. Most of these address global goals related to competencies expected at graduation and during subsequent practice. As such, they are essential for both teacher and learner. In most settings, they are well developed and regularly distributed to trainees. It is somewhat surprising therefore that one of students' and residents' most frequent complaints is that they do not know what is expected of them or the standard by which their performance will be judged.

To a large degree, the missing element is clarity about specifics. Students should already be aware that a goal of the rotation is for them to master diagnostic skills in that rotation's clinical area. What they most want to know is what time you expect them to come in, what information to present at rounds, and to whom their routine questions should be addressed. House officers understand that they will be evaluated on their patient care. They need to know what that means to you. Do you want them to check every order with you ahead of time? Do you want them to use lab tests liberally or conservatively? Do you prefer careful observation or aggressive treatment? To the degree that you are aware of your style compared to that of your colleagues, make it clear to your trainees.

The second complaint of residents is that they do not know how they are doing [17]. Give formative feedback regularly, including both positive and negative elements [18]. Give specific direction for improvement and follow-up feedback on the trainee's progress. Be sure your supervision includes the standards you will use in your summative assessment. There should never be a surprise when a student or resident reads a final evaluation.

Finally, trainees seek mentors more than supervisors [19]. Supervision is about direction, oversight, and evaluation. In the clinical setting, it is about ensuring that patient care meets appropriate standards and that trainees demonstrate appropriate skills. In several important ways, supervision is less about education than it is about the protection of patients in spite of education. Mentorship, in contrast, is a relationship between a trainee and a more experienced colleague who come together to share experience, knowledge, skills, and attitudes. A supervisor gives the trainee assignments; a mentor brings the trainee along as they work side by side on a common project. Supervisors give directions; mentors explain their thinking and invite the trainee to reason with them. Supervisors seek objectivity in evaluations; mentors seek a relationship that fosters growth. Supervision produces graduates; mentorship produces colleagues. Serve as a mentor by taking an interest in your students and residents, by inviting them into your professional world, by coming to know them as individuals, and by focusing your teaching less on the goals and objectives of the rotation and more on their goals as physicians.

The principle of mentorship applies equally well to relations between early-career and experienced faculty. As a new addition to the department, seek out senior people worthy of your trust and confidence. Ask them questions, seek their guidance, and learn from their experience. As you grow in experience, reach out to younger faculty, include them in your projects, share the insights you have gained, and try to help them move up the academic ladder. Treat their requests for your time and attention as the honor that they are. The relationships that result and the growth that follows will create a satisfying and productive work environment for early-career and experienced faculty alike.

Work Expectations and Schedules

One of the most frequently cited correlates with burnout among house officers and faculty is lack of control over schedules, work settings, and job expectations [12–14]. To the degree possible, seek residents' input in their rotation and call schedules and give faculty control over their daily schedules. Of course it will be necessary to set limits on their autonomy, but make clear the reasons those limits are set and how decisions are made. Once the schedule is in place, avoid unnecessary and last-minute changes. Constant and unpredictable changes in schedules are frustrating and demoralizing, enhancing the sense that their lives are out of their own control.

Monitor work expectations to ensure that they are reasonable. It is easy to achieve burnout among faculty simply by holding them accountable for 25 % more work than they can possibly do. The outcomes will be demoralization, cynicism, and exhaustion. Establish meaningful metrics of their work, such as hours, patients, or projects. Listen to their feedback on the viability of their workload. Spend time walking in their shoes, rotating through the clinics or completing a specific assignment. Make adjustments to keep things reasonable.

For trainees, the workload must be managed to avoid a compromise of the learning experience. Assignment of too few patients wastes their time and effort; assignment of too many deprives them of the opportunity to be thorough and reflective about what they are doing. Keep track of the numbers of hours they work, patients they see, and other work that they do. Seek their input regarding the value and burden of specific assignments. Make necessary adjustments promptly.

Social Activities

There is a reason that universities provide homes for their presidents and departments have catering budgets for their chairs [10]. Social gatherings are important to people who work together. In part, this is because eating, drinking, and socializing tend to be more fun than working. As such, receptions and parties can be ideal ways to thank people for their hard work or congratulate them on a recent achievement. Even a simple gift of food or flowers goes a long way to demonstrate recognition and appreciation.

The immediate effect of a social hour on morale is augmented by additional benefits. Some business is easier to conduct without a formal meeting, but other more global consequences are equally important. Opportunities to meet in a relaxed environment allow people to develop personal relationships that will assist them in the workplace. Informal meetings facilitate introductions across disciplines and along administrative hierarchies. Senior leaders usually seen at a podium or experienced only via mass-mailed communications become real and accessible people. New faculty members have faces and voices to accompany their names. Trainees stand equal ground with faculty as they chat together.

A good place to begin as a new faculty member is with bagels before rounds or cookies for a workroom. A word of explanation and a few minutes to share the snacks together will be appreciated as much as the food. Once or twice a year, consider hosting a picnic or theme party for trainees and their families. As you move up the administrative ladder, more formal gatherings may be appropriate. Take care to reach out to everyone within your sphere, including colleagues, trainees, and staff who might otherwise be overlooked. Develop the habit of social activity early. The benefits far exceed the costs.

Response to Complaints

No program or department is free of problems. Whether they are transient obstacles or long-term structural inadequacies, issues will periodically arise that cause dissatisfaction. The existence of these difficulties is less important than how they are handled [20]. Trainees and faculty want to be heard and respected when they call attention to a problem. They want to see some indication that their opinions make a difference. Morale may actually improve in the face of a challenge if people feel that they have a role in addressing it.

An effective leader welcomes feedback on the status of the workplace and quality of the work. Workers who care enough to confront a smoldering issue and offer an opinion about what is not working should be seen as an asset, not a liability. They may well hold the key to the problem and its solution.

Take seriously complaints from whatever source. Look into the problem to see if there is substance to it. If it cannot be objectively verified, try to understand why it is seen as a concern. Take action promptly to explore possible solutions. Engage those most affected in the process. Keep everyone apprised of what is going on. Make changes where you can; give explanations where you cannot (see Case Study #5).

Disaffected Personnel

A spirit of collegiality within a department can make the difference between a satisfying work experience and a tense, abrasive environment. One angry individual can stir up an entire program or department, often without it being immediately apparent where the trouble originated. In some cases, even the person who is agitating the situation is unaware of his or her role. Left uncorrected, the destructive influence of that individual on group cohesion and satisfaction can be devastating.

Your first obligation when an individual stirs up a group with complaints and angry dissatisfaction is to determine if this is a legitimate whistle-blower or if the person has become a scapegoat for a larger problem. A whistle-blower calls attention to an unacknowledged violation of legal requirements or local policies. A scapegoat is blamed for a systemic problem not of his or her making. A capable leader promptly recognizes and addresses the whistle-blower's concerns and helps to disentangle the scapegoated worker's role in the problem.

Once it has become clear that an individual is creating chaos and inappropriate concern within a group, several actions are appropriate. Make a sincere effort to understand the person's perspective. Promptly engage the rest of the group in the discussion to determine how widespread the concerns are. Educate everyone about the factors that led to the policy or situation about which some of them are angry. Seek their recommendations and act on the reasonable ones. Work to find common ground; avoid allowing the group to split into warring factions. If the problem persists, give the person at the center of the storm feedback on your view of his or her role. Throughout this process, your goal should be to bring the outlier back into the functioning group. Once that happens, things will calm down quickly.

Key Concepts
- Morale: the collective measure of job satisfaction, personal well-being, quality of interactions, and activity level of individuals that work together
- Engagement: recognition and acceptance of your responsibility as a leader, involvement with the people and processes with which you work, and active participation in decision-making
- Support: development of relationships that are respectful, warm, positive, and constructive, exemplified by empathic listening, emotional engagement, career assistance, and prompt feedback
- Transparency: clarity regarding goals and objectives, performance standards, decisions, and the processes by which they are established and monitored
- Direction and autonomy: the degree to which a person's work is directed by institutional versus individual priorities

Adverse Events and Disciplinary Action

Negative events are an unfortunate reality of academic medicine, whether they are related to unfavorable clinical outcomes, unsuccessful educational experiences, or transgression of regulatory expectations. These events require investigation, sometimes involve assignment of fault, may require corrective action such as remedial training or disciplinary sanctions, and may involve legal action. Because of the sensitive nature of the events that lead to these inquiries and the potential consequences of the findings, they are exceptionally difficult for the subject of the investigation, the investigator, and the administrative leader charged with deciding and implementing corrective action. Less well appreciated is the secondary impact of such action on the individual's peer group, who are likely to perceive the procedures not only as a problem for the subject of the action but as equally threatening to themselves.

Never underestimate the depth of vulnerability felt by students, house officers, and early-career faculty even under the best of circumstances. Insecure in their clinical skills and uncertain of their reputation among senior faculty, the prospect of their being found at fault and subjected to corrective action as a result of an adverse event or an administrative peccadillo can be overwhelming [5]. When the inevitable adverse event occurs, they fear the worst [21].

Transparency and support are the key elements of leadership when any investigation of clinical care becomes necessary. For routine adverse event reviews, make sure that the process and intent of the review are clear. Most trainees and even many faculty are unfamiliar with quality assurance procedures and assume that any review is about their performance. Take the time to explain the process, keep them informed about the findings, and above all, share the conclusions with them. Offer personal and professional support when appropriate. If the case is to be presented in a mortality and morbidity conference, ensure that it is done constructively. If there is a risk of legal action, involve risk management staff as early as possible.

Most cases of corrective action do not involve specific adverse events, but a failure to meet the expectations of a training program or faculty appointment. When this occurs, meet with the trainee or faculty member early and often through the process to explain exactly what is happening at each step. Offer support wherever possible, even if the outcome may be unfavorable. Consider the appointment of a faculty member to serve as advisor and advocate for the person during the case. Work to find the most constructive outcome for everyone involved. Give preferential consideration to remediation over termination. Even for the extreme case in which termination becomes unavoidable, do everything possible to establish a follow-up plan, such as a transfer to another program (with full disclosure to the receiving program), medical evaluation, additional training, or treatment, to address contributing factors. If someone has to walk the plank, make sure there is a lifeboat at the other end.

These extra actions are appropriate even in cases of egregious ethical violations, not least because of the collateral damage to morale that disciplinary actions can have on a program or department. Meet with residents and faculty periodically to go over the policies that govern corrective actions. When such action is contemplated, confidentiality prevents disclosure of details of the case, but a review of procedures will help allay fears of arbitrary, unfair, or disproportionate actions. Your attitude during these meetings conveys as much as the policies you present (see Case Study #6). Make clear that your goal is for every resident to successfully complete the program and for every faculty member to develop a flourishing career. Make sure your actions reflect that.

Conclusion

Morale requires the involvement of every person who works together, but there is much that a single individual can do, even from the bottom of the hierarchy. Awareness of self and others, constructive engagement, balance of direction with autonomy, and openness in decision-making and communication will set the stage for specific actions that contribute to a positive work environment and individual job satisfaction.

Words to the Wise
- As a supervisor and mentor, be supportive and transparent. Be clear in your expectations. Give prompt, specific, and constructive feedback. Share your experience and insights. Invite others to share in your work.
- Monitor trainee schedules and workloads to ensure that they are both manageable and constructive. Minimize noneducational service responsibilities (i.e., "scut work"). Be flexible about the amount of control you exercise over faculty job descriptions, giving as much autonomy as possible.
- Use social activities to build relationships, recognize accomplishments, and engender positive feelings.

(continued)

(continued)

- Be involved and supportive when handling complaints. Get those most affected by a problem engaged in finding a solution. Identify issues that can be corrected and move quickly to address them.
- Address difficult situations promptly, openly, and supportively. Be sensitive to those who have experienced untoward events. Use corrective action to help people succeed rather than to punish. Do your best to reintegrate those who are angry or discontent.

Ask Your Mentor or Colleagues

- What have been the hardest things for your students and residents to deal with? What have been the hardest things for the faculty?
- What things do the students and residents most value? What is most valued by faculty?
- What parts of your career have brought you the greatest satisfaction? Which parts the greatest frustration?
- What behind-the-scenes administrative issues (e.g., how work quality is judged, what it takes to get promoted, how adverse events are reviewed) most surprised you?
- How can I be most helpful to my colleagues and the department?
- How can I ensure that I have time to work on my most valued activities?

Appendix: Best Practices

Case Study #1

Dr. Beth Davidson, a second-year resident on a busy inpatient service, was in constant conflict with Linda, an experienced nurse on the service. Frustrated and angry by a recent caustic e-mail exchange, she sought out her attending to ask for help quashing the nurse. "Look at this sarcastic comment. You need to call her on the carpet for the way she is treating me." Dr. Rhoades, who had experienced a few of these communications himself in past years, chose a different approach. "Beth, I want you to take care of this yourself. You are responsible for the smooth operation of your team and who is at fault is less important than who will take the lead in fixing the problem. I will be interested to see how you handle it." A few days later, Dr. Davidson returned and excitedly reported, "I really had to bite my tongue, but I sat down with Linda and asked her to talk with me. She had some hard things to say about me and I did not agree with a lot of them, but I can see her point now. In the end, the only real change I needed to make was to give her a head's up before I wrote orders for her patients. I had no idea that was the problem."

Case Study #2

Dr. Wilkins was both excited and intimidated by his new role as program director. He loved teaching and had good relations with the residents he supervised. He quickly found, however, that the regulatory requirements of a residency program were daunting, especially with an accreditation site visit on the horizon. He soon found himself lost in administrative details and making decisions based on what looked good for the program rather than what was good for the residents. When the site visitor came, the files were in great shape, but the residents were not. They were all too anxious to share their dissatisfaction with the site visitor. "We never hear from Dr. Wilkins unless we are behind on our documentation, we have no idea how we are doing as residents, and no one seems to notice that we are here unless something goes wrong." Most of them said they were unhappy with the program and several wished they had gone elsewhere. The primary citations in the accreditation report were for poor engagement of the program director and low resident morale. In an effort to understand what was happening, Dr. Wilkins spent time over the next few weeks visiting residents on their clinical services, meeting with them after their lectures, and inviting them to his office for informal chats. Within a short time, before he implemented any other changes, morale was already improving.

Case Study #3

Dr. French was considering her options as she approached residency graduation. Always interested in community outreach and under-served populations, she hoped to find an outpatient position that would allow her to develop new clinic models to provide this service. Dr. Parker was the chair of a prominent research-oriented department that struggled to retain clinical staff, especially in its outpatient operation. With that in mind, he told Dr. French, "We have an opening in our outpatient clinic that we would like you to fill. With your interest in outreach, you should be able to do the work with no problem." Across town, Dr. Gage had a similar opening in a more modest department. After meeting with Dr. French to discuss her career interests, she said, "With your interest in outreach, a good place to start would be our outpatient clinic. With the experience you gain there, you will be well equipped to take the next step." Wanting an academic career, not just an academic job, Dr. French chose to forego prestige in favor of upward mobility and accepted Dr. Gage's offer.

Case Study #4

Dr. Norris enjoyed having medical students on his inpatient service. He found the opportunity to chat with them and hear their thinking about cases to be especially enjoyable. Dorothy, a third-year student, was anxious about the rotation. She had always been a bit awkward in social situations, and she found discussions in rounds especially trying. She tried to make up for this by studying hard and staying on top of every issue with her patients. Dr. Norris quickly noticed that Dorothy was not jumping in to answer questions and assumed that she was poorly prepared. Preferring the livelier interactions with the other students, Dr. Norris stopped calling on Dorothy, who experienced relief to be out of the limelight. Not having heard that anything was wrong, Dorothy was taken aback to receive an evaluation that said she had a poor fund of knowledge and seemed disengaged from clinical care. Her evaluation of Dr. Norris complained that she was never told there was a problem or given the opportunity to improve things. Taking this evaluation to heart, Dr. Norris began to give feedback promptly and frequently, and soon noticed a sharp improvement in students' performance and his own evaluations.

Case Study #5

Dr. Logan had worked hard to ensure that recent changes in ACGME work hours did not disrupt her residents' educational experience or clinical care. Her plan to create a senior resident night float and limit PGY-1 residents to the inpatient day shift seemed the perfect arrangement to stay within the guidelines. She was taken aback, then, to learn that both the interns and the senior residents felt overburdened and unhappy with the experience. Her initial response was anger at their complaints, and she planned to confront them with work-hour reports to show how much less they were working than previous classes. Instead, what she heard when she met with them changed her mind. They pointed out that most admissions to the inpatient unit came in late in the afternoon and were directed to the night float, placing most of the assessment and planning for new patients in the hands of the senior residents and leaving the interns to implement the plans the following day. Consequently, the senior residents felt like they were "on call every night" and the interns felt overwhelmed by "scut work" of little educational value. They did not want fewer hours but more direct involvement with the new patients and suggested a rotating "short-call" assignment alongside the senior residents. This would allow them to perform more patient assessments and plans and would change the senior residents' role to teacher and supervisor. Dr. Logan made a few phone calls to affected faculty and implemented the change the following month. The residents commented that the responsiveness of their training director to their concerns was as important to them as the change in job description.

Case Study #6

Dr. Carter was a popular and capable third-year resident, with a roguish disdain for meaningless bureaucracy. Though attentive to his patients, he was openly defiant about treatment plans, billing forms, and insurance reviews. Despite repeated reminders and warnings, he refused to complete this paperwork until a major payor threatened to terminate its relationship with the clinic because of noncompliance with these requirements. The program director, Dr. Walters, was finally forced to convene a disciplinary hearing. Morale plummeted as Dr. Carter stirred up his colleagues over the issue. Bound by confidentiality rules regarding the hearing, Dr. Walters could not share the details of the case but arranged a meeting of the residency class to explain the rationale for the documentation requirements, the procedures that had been followed before the hearing, who was on the hearing committee, and the mechanics of the disciplinary process. One member of the class commented afterward, "Dr. Walters did not really tell us anything about Dr. Carter's case, but we felt a lot better knowing what was going on behind the scenes."

References

1. McCray LW, Cronholm PF, Bogner HR, et al. Resident physician burnout: is there hope? Fam Med. 2008;40:626–32.
2. Williams ES, Skinner AC. Outcomes of physician job satisfaction: a narrative review, implications, and directions for future research. Health Care Manage Rev. 2003;28:119–39.
3. Klann G. Building your team's morale, pride, and spirit. Greensboro, NC: Center for Creative Leadership; 2004.

4. Van Ham I, Verhoeven AA, Groenier KH, et al. Job satisfaction among general practitioners: a systematic literature review. Eur J Gen Prac. 2006;12:174–80.
5. Yeo H, Viola K, Berg D, et al. Attitudes, training experiences, and professional expectations of US general surgery residents: a national survey. JAMA. 2009;302:1301–8.
6. Ellencweig N, Weizman A, Fischel T. Factors determining satisfaction in psychiatry training in Israel. Acad Psychiatry. 2009;33:169–73.
7. Munro S. Balance, safety, and passion: three principles for academic leaders. Acad Psychiatry. 2011;35:134–5.
8. Tasman A. Reminiscences and reflections on leadership. Acad Psychiatry. 2011;35:129–33.
9. Keith SJ, Buckley PF. Leadership experiences and characteristics of chairs of academic departments of psychiatry. Acad Psychiatry. 2011;35:118–21.
10. Winstead D. Advice for chairs of academic departments of psychiatry: the ten commandments. Acad Psychiatry. 2006;30:298–300.
11. Scott G. Leading in hard times: successful strategies to ensure employee commitment and loyalty in times of change. Healthc Exec. 2009;24(3):60–3.
12. Keeton K, Fenner DE, Johnson TRB, Hayward RA. Predictors of physician career satisfaction, work–life balance, and burnout. Obstet Gynecol. 2007;109:949–55.
13. Scheurer D, McKean S, Miller J, Wetterneck T. U.S. physician satisfaction: a systematic review. J Hosp Med. 2009;4:560–8.
14. Shanafelt TD, West CP, Sloan JA, et al. Career fit and burnout among academic faculty. Arch Intern Med. 2009;169:990–5.
15. Souba WW, Mauger D, Day DV. Does agreement on institutional values and leadership issues between deans and surgery chairs predict their institutions' performance? Acad Med. 2007;82:272–80.
16. Cannon GW, Keitz SA, Holland GJ, et al. Factors determining medical students' and residents' satisfaction during VA-based training: findings from the VA Learners' Perceptions Survey. Acad Med. 2008;83:611–20.
17. Gil DH, Heins M, Jones PB. Perceptions of medical school faculty members and students on clinical clerkship feedback. J Med Educ. 1984;59:856–64.
18. Ende J. Feedback in clinical medical education. JAMA. 1983;250:777–81.
19. Cho CS, Ramanan RA, Feldman MD. Defining the ideal qualities of mentorship: a qualitative analysis of the characteristics of outstanding mentors. Am J Med. 2011;124:453–8.
20. Freeman SR, Greene RE, Kimball AB, et al. US dermatology residents' satisfaction with training and mentoring: survey results from the 2005 and 2006 Las Vegas Dermatology Seminars. Arch Dermatol. 2008;143:896–900.
21. Fang F, Kemp J, Jawandha A, et al. Encountering patient suicide: a resident's experience. Acad Psychiatry. 2007;31:340–4.

How to Network and Be a Good Colleague

15

Edward Kass and Laura B. Dunn

At first blush, "how to network" and "how to be a good colleague" may seem like disparate topics. However, there is substantial overlap between them. They both involve attending thoughtfully and genuinely to the relationships that pervade our professional and personal lives. Both involve considering others' needs and our own. Moreover, learning the skills and habits to network well and be a good colleague hold immense potential to improve the quality of our lives—and our connections to one another—in academic medicine.

Our relationships with others have strong effects on our well-being and that of our colleagues and patients. The importance of the physician–patient relationship is exemplified in the model of relationship-centered care (RCC), which was proposed in 2006 as a reframing of clinical care beyond "patient-centered care" to a model anchored in values and relationships. The principles of RCC focus strongly on relationships—not only those of physicians with their patients but also the interactions physicians have

E. Kass, Ph.D. (✉)
Department of Organization, Leadership, and Communication,
University of San Francisco, School of Management, 2130 Fulton Street,
San Francisco, CA, USA
e-mail: ekass@usfca.edu

© Springer International Publishing Switzerland 2016
L.W. Roberts (ed.), *The Associate Professor Guidebook*,
DOI 10.1007/978-3-319-28001-1_15

with one another [1]. Regarding collegial relationships, the RCC model states:

> Relationship-centered care recognizes that the relationships that clinicians form with each other, especially within hierarchical organizations, contribute meaningfully to their own well-being as well as the health of patients….Relationship-centered care emphasizes that clinicians ought to listen, respect colleagues, appreciate the contributions that colleagues from other disciplines bring, promote sincere teamwork, bridge differences, and learn from and celebrate the accomplishments of their colleagues.

Further evidence recognizing the value of collegial relationships comes from the Institute of Medicine's report *Improving Medical Education: Enhancing the Behavioral and Social Science Content of Medical School Curricula*, which rated learning to work in teams and organizations and physician well-being as high priorities for medical school curricula [2].

Thus, the topics addressed in this chapter have direct relevance not only to our professional lives and personal well-being but also to those whose lives we touch.

Networking

Networks—whether defined as one's network of friends, family, and colleagues or permutations of all three—can serve to support and promote our personal and professional needs while fostering a greater sense of connectedness and responsibility within our community. The term "social network" has taken on added meaning with the advent of internet-based networking. Here, we use the term "social network" to encompass the entirety of one's contacts, both personal and professional.

In academic medicine, our social networks—if tended to thoughtfully—can be a primary source of social support, satisfaction, and personal and professional development. Moreover, these networks are strongly associated with scientific creativity, job performance, finding new jobs, and promotion. In addition to driving individual development and success, social networks are also associated with departmental and even organizational success.

Despite the large impact of social networks, many in academic medicine feel uncomfortable with "networking." We may have unexamined assumptions about what networking means—perhaps associating the term with insincerity, using other people for one's own gain, or other negative connotations. If we do recognize the utility of networking, we may feel that we do not know how to network or that we do not network as much as we could or even as much as we believe we "should." This is unfortunate, for several reasons. First, those who are uncomfortable with networking and developing the power of their network may misunderstand what constitutes "effective networking" and how "social networks" affect their members—and therefore may be missing out on important opportunities. Second, those who are more uncomfortable with networking may be precisely those individuals who should network more—in other words, lack of networking may reinforce avoidant tendencies and may become a self-fulfilling prophecy of relative isolation. Third, failure to network has costs, which, though difficult to measure, are nevertheless important to our individual and collective success.

The need for improved use of the positive aspects of our networks has never been greater. Recent research on peak and frustrating experiences of academic physicians revealed that relationships were a central theme in respondents' descriptions of their most satisfying and frustrating experiences in academic medicine [3]. Using qualitative interview methods, the authors reported that faculty who discussed their most frustrating experiences tended to identify a lack of supportive relationships, feeling socially isolated, not being recognized as a person beyond her or his professional work role, disrespect and mistrust or low trust, and the negative effects of "competitive individualism." On the other hand, faculty who discussed peak experiences linked them with positive relationships, emotional support, a sense of belonging, and collaboration. Positive aspects of relationships with colleagues illustrated the support and connection that networks can provide. For example, one of the senior women interviewed expressed both her lack of overall connectedness within her institution and the importance of the research group itself to her sense of belonging: "I felt very little of a sense of belonging except to my own research

group, which felt like a team with a wonderful mix of people."
Another early-career faculty member described his feeling of isolation by stating:

> "I couldn't pick out anybody that I corresponded with by e-mail or let-
> ters out of a line-up. I knew very few people in different divisions. It
> was very much an isolated situation. Go to your clinic, do your thing,
> go back to your office, go to the medical suite, do your procedures, go
> back to the office."

The authors of this study concluded that disconnectedness is a
major challenge in academic medicine and recommended that
institutions work to improve "relational practices in medical
schools," with putative beneficial effects on communication and
collaboration in all of the core missions of medical schools, as well
as "a more satisfied and energized faculty."

Another recent study found substantial levels of depression,
anxiety, and job dissatisfaction among medical school faculty,
although overall life satisfaction was high [4]. The authors were
particularly concerned about findings of higher levels of depression and anxiety among younger faculty. Taken together, such
findings underscore the need for greater attention to the relationships that support, promote, and nurture the current and future
generations of academic medicine faculty. Effective networking is
one way that individuals can work to bolster their sense of belonging and foster greater connection among their colleagues.
Moreover, institutions can and should work harder to help faculty
develop broader networks of ties with one another, in turn fostering greater institutional cohesion and morale.

Effective networking does not mean collecting as many business cards, phone numbers, or online friends or connections as
possible. It does not mean being inauthentic or viewing others
instrumentally or in an objectified fashion. It does not have to substitute for performance but, rather, can become a tool for performing well.

An entire field of social network analysis examines how social
networks operate [5]. However, most in academic medicine remain
unaware of this field, its findings, or its implications for effective
networking. Social network scholars view an individual as

Key Concepts
- Social networks: The social structure of a group, comprising the individuals and the relationships (or lack of relationships) between them.
- The power of weak ties: The finding that people are more likely to get help from weak relationships than strong ones.
- Relationship-centered care: Care in which central principles and values are focused on relationships, i.e., between patient and clinician, among clinicians themselves, and between clinicians and themselves [1].
- Positive "no": A "no" sandwiched between two "yes's" or other affirmative statements.

embedded in a larger web of relationships. In this web, a node represents each individual, and the lines connecting nodes represent the ties or relationships between individuals. These ties can be strong or weak and can be of various kinds, for example, friendship networks (who likes whom) or advice networks (who goes to whom for advice). In this way, a social network can be mapped and made visible. As shown in Fig. 15.1, our social networks are the context in which each of us is embedded.

Networks provide social support. They also affect one's professional life. In one of the seminal studies in social network analysis, Granovetter explored whether people tended to get new jobs from job postings or through informal social networks and whether jobs were found primarily through stronger relationships or weaker ones [6]. The main finding was that most people found their jobs through informal relationships. Another finding was that the strength of the relationship also mattered. Surprisingly, Granovetter found that people were far more likely to get jobs through weak ties rather than strong ones. This is a key finding for understanding how "weak ties" in social networks can translate into important opportunities in academic medicine.

We share information with those in our network. And new information is a primary mediator through which social networks

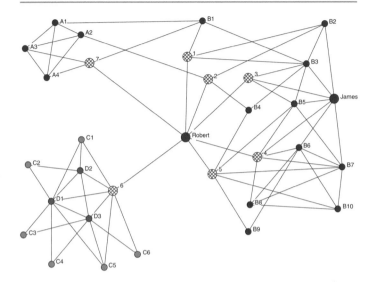

Fig. 15.1 Example of a social network: *circles* people, *lines* relationships. Reprinted with permission from Burt RS: Brokerage and Closure: An introduction to social capital. Oxford University Press, 2007

translate into results. For instance, one may learn new and critical information that will only be available to others at a later date, such as that a job will be available in a given department or specialty in approximately 3 months but that this information will not be made public until then. Even more beneficial is knowing about an opening in a given clinic or hospital ahead of time—even before the job duties and requirements have been finalized, when one can help negotiate the job requirements to match one's skills and background.

If social networks are the key to information, why is cultivating "weak ties" important? Further research in social networks discovered that it was not the weakness, per se, that caused the advantage. It was something that tended to correlate with weakness—diversity [7, 8]. Our tendency is to like people who remind us of ourselves. This "similar to me" effect is a widely studied phenomenon in social psychology [9, 10]. Internists, pediatricians, surgeons, and psychiatrists—we tend to stick together and feel more comfortable with our colleagues most similar to us. This may be even more of an issue in medicine than has been documented, because of increased specialization.

Left unchecked, however, this tendency can cause us to limit our strong ties (and perhaps all of our ties) to overly similar others. This is problematic in academic medicine because we tend to know the same people, read the same journals, and have access to similar information. Even though we may be motivated to help one another, our "help" may not be very helpful. If your network largely comprises people who are very similar to you, they are unlikely to have information that is new to you.

The key to enhancing the benefits of one's network for problem solving and performance is diversity. Access to new and different information enhances creativity. Sometimes creative solutions are developed by importing something (e.g., information or a proce-dure) that is common in one domain into another domain in which it has not been used. For example, medical education may draw on leadership principles that are common in the fields of organiza-tional behavior or organizational development to create physician leadership programs that are novel and effective in the medical domain. Organizational scholarship was enhanced by applying open systems models from biology to organizations.

Diverse networks can also lead to creativity when one brings together unconnected information in new ways. Dr. Deborah Rhodes' development of gamma mammography exemplifies this type of creativity [11]. She had an identified problem, the high error rate in X-ray mammography interpretation. Rhodes met a nuclear physicist, Michael O'Connor, who mentioned that he had just returned from a conference in Israel where someone had reported a new type of gamma detector. The new detector was manufactured through a completely different process and could be made very small. Rhodes knew that breast density is strongly asso-ciated with X-ray mammography interpretation error-rates and that gamma detectors are not influenced by breast density. But gamma detectors have not been very useful in detecting breast can-cer because of their size and bulkiness. She wondered if the new detector would be usable for mammography. Rhodes, an internist, and O'Connor, a nuclear physicist, along with a biomedical engineer, two radiologists, and some duct tape, were able to develop and test the molecular breast imaging machine (MBI), which has now been demonstrated to work extremely effectively with high density breast tissue.

There are two complementary ways of looking at diversity. One is to directly look at your network members. To whom are you connected? To what extent does your network have diversity or manifest homogeneity? Another approach is to look at the map of the larger network structure. This method is particularly important for accessing information that others do not have. If you are connected to people who are also highly connected with one another, you all probably share a lot of the same information. If you are connected to people or groups of people who are not otherwise connected to others in your network, you are in a brokerage position. This position will provide you with more opportunities and more information that is not shared by others. Practically, this also means that you are more likely to be seen as an "opinion leader."

Networks may be even more important for women and minorities in academic medicine. Women in academia tend to experience more social isolation [12–14], which negatively affects career progression. But everyone can benefit by paying attention to networks, increasing the diversity of the networks, and enhancing the ties within these networks.

How can you increase the diversity in your network? By being authentically curious about others. People are interesting. And if you learn more about them, you are more likely to learn something about them that you like. You are also more likely to identify something that you share in common. We already mentioned the "similar to me" effect. People like people who are seen as similar to themselves. However, the "similar to me" effect is perceptual; it does not take very much to induce a feeling of similarity. if you discover something that you and another person share in common, this similarity, however small, is likely to cause both of you to like each other more. In this way, the "similar to me" effect can be harnessed to increase diversity in a network by building trust and liking among people who are dissimilar in many ways by finding something (e.g., hobby, interest, and attitude) shared in common. However, feigning similarity is ill-advised: although it may increase another person's liking for you, it will do nothing positive for your liking of him or her. You may even like the person less for believing your falsehood. That said, it is usually not too difficult to find something in common with others.

Woody Allen famously said that 80 % of success is just showing up. You need to be visible and interact with others in order to build relationships with them. Increasing your visibility keeps you "top of mind" for others. When someone discovers information or opportunities that would be relevant for you, that person needs to remember the relevance or will not do anything about it. Visibility also matters because people like what is familiar, the mere exposure effect [15]. Being seen more often makes you more familiar and thereby increases liking. Finally, visibility and frequency of interaction provide the opportunity to develop relationships with others and to build a reputation.

A famous study at MIT found that functional distance on a dormitory hall was a powerful predictor of friendships [16]. People were 41 % likely to be friends with their next-door neighbor. The likelihood of friendship dropped by almost half for those living two doors away and to 10 % for those living four doors away. More recently, Lee and colleagues studied the relationship between physical distance apart among Harvard biomedical researchers and the effect on publications [17]. They found an inverse relationship between the actual distance between the first and last author and the mean number of citations of their publications.

physical space and distance continue to matter, despite the ubiquity of technologies that make it easy to work together over distance. So, engage in activities that bring you into greater proximity to colleagues and potential colleagues or collaborators. Going to conferences, joining special interest groups, and volunteering your time all provide activities in which you are likely to meet others and engage meaningfully. By trying something new, you are also more likely to meet interesting others who are different from you. Meeting people while engaging in activities is also helpful because it allows you to interact in a way that enhances the likelihood of learning about another as a unique human being rather than as an object. How many people do you see regularly? Who are they? And what do they see when they see you?

Exchanging favors is a powerful way of building relationships with others. Helping others requires thought about others' interests and what would help them, which builds the habit of seeing others as people rather than objects. attempting to thoughtfully help others sends a signal that you care about their well-being. Helping others also elicits reciprocity, a desire to respond in kind [18].

We have two caveats regarding favors and mutualism. First, do not downplay favors. How many times have you responded to a strong and sincere thank you from someone else by saying, "It was nothing"? How many times have you said it was nothing when, in fact, doing the favor entailed real effort? If the favor really required no additional effort, by all means say so. However, if effort was required, you are shortchanging yourself by discounting your effort on the other's behalf. Even worse, you, in effect, signal that you were not concerned about the other's well-being; you merely helped because it was easy to do so. This is the wrong message to send and can undermine relationship building. Instead, a brief "It was my pleasure to help," or "Happy I could help you out" is more genuine in demonstrating your underlying motivation. Second, although reciprocal favors often ensue, they should not be expected.

Being a Good Colleague

Nice is different than good.

Stephen Sondheim

We receive many messages in academic medicine, including the message to be a "good citizen" within our department and institution. Does being a "good citizen" entail being "nice"? This confusion between "nice" and "good" may be one of the seeds of disillusionment. In the study cited earlier, a lack of recognition for the daily work of academic medicine was mentioned as a negative aspect of professional life by an early-career woman physician:

> We're not rewarded by the medical school at all. We're not recognized. A few people each year might be recognized, but for the ongoing day-to-day grind, we're not recognized by the medical school for our efforts [3].

Thus, while many in academic medicine feel a great deal of pressure to meet some standard for being a "good citizen" or "good colleague," there may be a knowledge gap in understanding what these standards entail. Some try hard to be "good" by, in essence, being "nice"—e.g., by volunteering for many committees, taking on numerous clinical duties, shouldering heavy teaching responsibilities, or taking on more in writing or editorial responsibilities than one can realistically handle. If these tasks begin to feel like more than one's fair share of citizenship, they can lead to burnout, resentment, and disillusionment. Therefore, it is worthwhile to get clarity on what it means to be a "good" colleague.

Increasing the diversity of your network does not mean that you will blindly build relationships with everyone, nor even everyone who is different than you. If someone demonstrates that he or she is untrustworthy or unpleasant, you may choose to not build a relationship with that person. To what kinds of colleagues are we most suited to being "good" colleagues? This kind of reflection means being honest with ourselves. Personal experiences may have taught us that some colleagues may just rub us the wrong way or treat us disrespectfully or be manipulative or even dishonest.

We do not need to "force" a relationship that we know is not going to work, and we need to listen to our instincts. It is important to find mentors and collaborators whose work and team style mesh well with our own and to acknowledge that it is fine to *not* want to work with everyone and to say no to collaborations or other collegial activities that we know will not be productive, will be psychologically unhealthy (e.g., an abusive colleague), or will otherwise be too stressful. "Going along to get along" in spite of our reservations may be at the root of many of the difficulties we encounter or witness in academia. Therefore, being a good colleague does not involve subjecting oneself to harmful situations or even situations that are less than satisfying, simply for the sake of some notion of "harmony." This may go against the ways that some of us were socialized to behave; however, it is fundamental to healthy relationships with others and ourselves to heed one's better judgment, including listening to nagging doubts. When in doubt, seek out a trusted friend or confidante with whom to discuss these issues before jumping into, or ending, a work relationship.

Similarly, we have recommended engaging in favors. However, this does not mean that you should say yes to every request. Saying yes and saying no are equally important. saying yes to a committee assignment, clinical or teaching duty, or research collaboration simply to be nice is a recipe for resentment. If others fail to recognize and value your favors, you may choose to say no. Saying no when you lack the interest or time to invest and do a good job is not only good; it is the right thing to do. Your colleague will be better off having a teammate or collaborator who can put in the needed effort. If you say yes when you do not have the time or resources, you are likely to fail to follow through and thus develop a reputation for unreliability, not helpfulness. See Table 15.1 for tips on saying yes and saying no.

If you realize you have simply agreed to too many obligations, it is better to let your colleague know sooner rather than later, in fairness to the other person. Waiting until later leaves the colleague with even less time before the deadline to make up the work that you have chosen to not do. Avoiding a difficult conversation simply puts the other person in a tougher position later. If at all possible, find someone who can fill in for you in the task.

If you have a colleague who is asking things of you that you feel are unreasonable (e.g., to edit a manuscript with a 2-day turn-around time), you need to speak up—for your own sake and your colleague's. Being clear and straightforward—and leaving out any associated emotions—is the best way to address these situations. For example, here is some wording to handle the urgent or quick-turnaround request:

> "I am eager to read your manuscript and appreciate your asking for my thoughts on this. However, it is important to me that I do a good job in my responses so they can be most useful to you. I would need a week to get this back to you, due to my other obligations. I had a couple of thoughts about how we could handle this: one would be that I go ahead and send you my comments by the end of next week; the other option would be for me not to take this on at this time. I would be more than happy to look at a later draft. Let me know what you would prefer."

Table 15.1 Tips for saying "yes" and saying "no"

Saying "yes"
Be enthusiastic about new roles or duties when you do accept them (no one wants a grudging commitment)
Indicate your desire to do a good job (no one wants a colleague who is saying "yes" but does not intend to do their best.) Even though you may think that this goes without saying, it does not
Be clear *why* you are saying "yes," as this can be an opportunity to strengthen relationships and indicate your interests and your desire to help others (e.g., "I enjoy working with you." "I liked our previous collaboration a lot." "I know I will learn a lot about [X] while working on this." "I enjoy working on these issues with others who care about them.")
Discuss any limits up front and negotiate these when necessary (e.g., if you need additional time, want to enlist a coauthor, etc.)
Saying "no"
Saying "no" with no explanation can appear abrupt or rude
Saying "no" but being clear *why* one needs to say "no" is likely to be respected
When saying "no" to specific requests (e.g., manuscript reviews), consider whether this may be an opportunity to help a colleague (e.g., suggest a colleague with appropriate expertise who might be able to review the manuscript, and who may need some scholarly activities.)
Saying "no" to obligations that one cannot fulfill is appropriate and helps your colleagues. When possible, try to identify an appropriate alternative
If there are conditions that might turn your "no" into a "yes," ask about these. The other person may not have considered these possibilities, but might be grateful for your creativity. For example, a writing assignment may be more feasible, and more fun, if you enlist a colleague or a mentee

Colleagues and Life Balance Issues

We all have times when it is wholly appropriate to invoke our "life" as in need of care and feeding, including setting limits on new obligations—e.g., not accepting work with urgent deadlines prior to leaving on vacation.

William Ury, the negotiator and author of *Getting to Yes*, has written in *The Power of a Positive No* that the key to saying no effectively is respect [19]. This idea sounds simple, but it can be very challenging to deliver a respectful "no" that does not hurt or offend. Ury does an excellent job describing the components and skills needed to use "no" effectively and to maintain relationships in the process.

In developing strong and trusting relationships with colleagues, much of the advice on networking applies: Stay in touch. Be genuine. Be curious. Basic courtesy is also critical. But most important, be trustworthy. If someone confides in you, do not use that information to gain an advantage. the benefits of being trustworthy in the work setting far outweigh any perceived benefits of being "strategic" in manipulative ways.

Finally, development of a network of trusted colleagues can make all the difference between a fulfilling career where great satisfaction comes from our work relationships and a job that one is eager to leave each day. Being a good colleague to others will bring its own rewards.

Supporting Your Colleagues in Their Careers

Being a good colleague also means looking for opportunities to help your colleagues advance. You can nominate people for awards and recognition within your institution and in local, regional, national, and international organizations. It is quite an honor to be recognized by one's peers as deserving of these awards. Look for opportunities to nominate people who have not received recognition already but who are clearly excelling in their work.

Other opportunities exist to help your colleagues—such as by suggesting their names as speakers, teachers, administrators, or collaborators for any number of projects. This fits in nicely with the concepts of saying no in a positive way: "I would love to help you out with this chapter. However, I am overcommitted right now. But I do have a colleague who I think would do a great job on this."

Clearly, one of the most common requests in academic medicine is for help for another colleague's relatives, friends, or neighbors with medical issues, questions, or referrals. Curbside consultations, requests to "squeeze in" new patients, and even urgent calls asking for help are commonplace. Clearly, these requests can put the academic clinician in a very difficult situation on several levels — personally (by taking up precious time), professionally (by putting pressure on the academician and sometimes by challenging the limits of competencies), as well as ethically (by seeking favors that allow well-connected people to "jump the line" for clinical care). When possible, offer help within your comfort zone of competence, offer referrals to clinicians in whose skills you feel confident, or simply try to provide a positive no if you truly cannot help at that time. clarify that while you are happy to brainstorm quickly, you are not always available to solve complicated problems or take on new clinical responsibilities.

Being a good colleague, then, involves knowing oneself, knowing one's limits and traits, and working with those optimally, with appropriate boundaries, in one's interactions with colleagues.

Ironically, those who are focused on instrumentally "networking" tend to behave in ways that cause them to lose network benefits. Networking by developing an interest in others and growing authentic relationships with colleagues supports the individual and the network. The more that one thoughtfully gives to one's network through social support and diverse information and skills and greater creativity, the more benefits that one (and one's network) reaps. Many of the biases that can disrupt powerful networks (e.g., the "similar to me" effect) can be avoided and even harnessed to increase diversity and authentic relationships rather than minimize them. The key is to be authentic and to care, both about others and for oneself.

Words to the Wise
- Be passionate.
- Be sincere and genuine.
- Be curious about others and demonstrate your interest.
- Expect the best and see the best in others.
- Identify nonobvious similarities with others.
- Seek out diversity.
- Engage in a variety of activities.
- Committees
- Grand rounds

(continued)

(continued)
- Interacting with others you might not otherwise contact.
- Help others and do favors (and don't discount these).
- Accept help and favors from others (even small ones).
- Every interaction is an opportunity to demonstrate trust-worthiness and reliability.
- Keep in touch with others.

Ask Your Mentor or Colleagues
- What have been the most effective ways you have found to network?
- What organizations have you joined and what has been your experience with those?
- Where/how would you suggest I consider looking, if I am trying to diversify my network?
- What skills and qualities do you find most/least helpful in your colleagues and collaborators?
- What do you find most satisfying/least satisfying in your day-to-day work relationships? What would you suggest as ways to improve those relationships?
- Have you had any experiences that you found to be particularly good/bad for networking? Why? What would you have done differently?

References

1. Beach MC, Inui T. Relationship-centered care. A constructive reframing. J Gen Intern Med. 2006;21 Suppl 1:S3–8.
2. Cuff PA, Vanselow, N (Eds). Committee on Behavioral and Social Sciences in Medical School Curricula. Improving Medical Education: Enhancing the Behavioral and Social Science Content of Medical School Curricula. Washington DC: The National Academies Press; 2004.
3. Pololi L, Conrad P, Knight S, et al. A study of the relational aspects of the culture of academic medicine. Acad Med. 2009;84:106–14.

4. Schindler BA, Novack DH, Cohen DG, et al. The impact of the changing health care environment on the health and well-being of faculty at four medical schools. Acad Med. 2006;81:27–34.

5. Borgatti SP, Mehra A, Brass DJ, et al. Network analysis in the social sciences. Science. 2009;323:892–5.

6. Granovetter M. The strength of weak ties. Am J Sociol. 1973;78: 1360–80.

7. Granovetter M. The strength of weak ties: a network theory revisited. In: Marsden P, Lin N, editors. Social structure and network analysis. New York: John Wiley and Sons; 1982. p. 105–30.

8. Burt RS. Structural holes: the social structure of competition. Boston: Harvard University; 1992.

9. Montoya RM, Horton RS, Kirchner J. Is actual similarity necessary for attraction? A meta-analysis of actual and perceived similarity. J Soc Pers Relat. 2008;25:889–922.

10. Byrne D. The attraction paradigm. London: Academic; 1971.

11. Deborah Rhodes: a tool that finds 3x more breast tumors, and why it's not available to you. 2011. http://www.ted.com/talks/deborah_rhodes.html . Accessed Jan 6 2011.

12. Reskin B. Sex differentiation and the social organization of science. In: Gaston J, editor. Sociology of science. San Francisco: Jossey Bass; 1978. p. 6–37.

13. Epstein C. Woman's place: options and limits in professional careers. Berkeley: University of California; 1970.

14. Emmett A. A woman's institute of technology. Technol Rev. 1992; April: 16–8.

15. Bornstein RF. Exposure and affect: overview and meta-analysis of research, 1968–1987. Psychological Bulletin. 1989;106:265–289.

16. Festinger L, Schachter S, Back K. Social pressures in informal groups: a study of human factors in housing. Palo Alto, CA: Stanford University; 1950.

17. Lee K, Brownstein JS, Mills RG, et al. Does collocation inform the impact of collaboration? PLoS One. 2010;5:e14279.

18. Gouldner AW. The norm of reciprocity: a preliminary statement. Am Sociol Rev. 1960;25:161–78.

19. Ury W. The power of a positive no. New York: Bantam Books; 2007.

How to Recognize and Address Unconscious Bias

16

Daisy Grewal, Manwai Candy Ku,
Sabine C. Girod, and Hannah Valantine

Despite the dramatic increase in the number of women and racial minorities pursuing careers in medicine, their representation among medical school faculty remains strikingly low. One potential explanation for this disparity is *unconscious bias*: opinions that we hold about different social groups that operate outside of our conscious awareness. During the past few decades, social scientists have discovered that unconscious bias can strongly influence the way we evaluate and treat other people. For that reason, it is important to understand what unconscious bias is and how it might influence one's career.

The medical field has become increasingly diverse in the past 49 years. Women now make up half of all medical school students. The number of racial minorities in medical school has also increased: between 2010 and 2011, enrollment grew by 9 % among Hispanics, 2.9 % among African-Americans, and 24.8 % among Native American students. Despite these changes, a 2010 report by the Association of American Medical Colleges (AAMC) found that women and minorities make up a small proportion of faculty in

H. Valantine, M.D. (✉)
Department of Office of Diversity and Leadership/Cardiovascular Medicine, Stanford University School of Medicine,
291 Campus Drive, Stanford, CA, USA
e-mail: hvalantine@stanford.edu

© Springer International Publishing Switzerland 2016
L.W. Roberts (ed.), *The Associate Professor Guidebook*,
DOI 10.1007/978-3-319-28001-1_16

academic medicine. According to AAMC estimates, women make up only 35 % of all medical school faculty and just 19 % of faculty at the rank of Full Professor. African-Americans and those of Hispanic origin make up only about 7 % of all medical school faculty. The composition of medical school faculty has not kept up with either the growing diversity of physicians-in-training or society at large.

Enough time has passed such that "pipeline" explanations cannot explain these disparities. In fact, the data for women's career advancement in academic medicine show greater resemblance to a funnel than a pipeline (see Fig. 16.1). We believe that until individuals and institutions address the issue of unconscious bias, faculty from underrepresented groups will continue to have a difficult time climbing the academic ladder. The aim of this chapter is to help the academic physician identify and understand unconscious bias so that he or she may take steps to prevent it from negatively influencing his or her career.

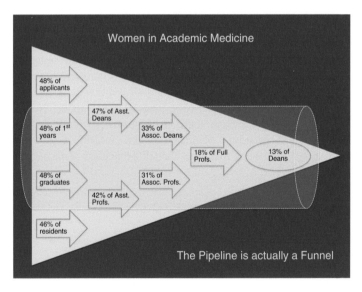

Fig. 16.1 The career advancement of women in academic medicine resembles a funnel rather than a pipeline

What Is Unconscious Bias?

Unconscious bias includes opinions and attitudes that we are not consciously aware of having. Unconscious bias can be difficult to grasp because it contradicts what we intuitively believe about human behavior: we tend to think that most of our behavior and our thoughts are intentional and chosen. However, social scientists have found that thoughts and feelings outside of our conscious awareness have the power to influence us in important ways. Although we can hold unconscious biases about anything or anyone, this chapter focuses on the biases we hold about people from underrepresented social groups. For example, many people hold an unconscious bias that men are more likely than women to have an aptitude for science. In the psychology research literature, the terms *implicit attitude* or *implicit bias* are often used interchangeably with *unconscious bias*.

Where do our unconscious biases come from? Why do we have them? Psychologists believe that unconscious bias results from the way in which our brains process and store information. Research from cognitive psychology has shown that all of us use mental shortcuts in order to quickly process new information about the world. One of these shortcuts is automatically sorting people into categories such as age, gender, and race. Categorizing others in this way helps us quickly determine how to interact with people with whom we are not familiar.

Using mental shortcuts is not necessarily a bad thing. Without them we would be paralyzed by the amount of information that we receive from the outside world. Physicians often use mental shortcuts in order to make quick and efficient diagnoses of patients in time-pressured situations. However, mental shortcuts become a problem when they lead to s*tereotyping*—when we make assumptions about an individual based on what we think members of that person's social group are like. Stereotyping may lead us to treat people in unfair and unjustified ways. Many people believe that stereotypes do not influence their opinions about others. Regardless, numerous studies show that stereotypes can enter our minds without us being fully aware of them. This means that we can end up stereotyping others even when we have a strong desire not to.

This *unconscious stereotyping* occurs because of our tendency to automatically sort people into categories. When we encounter somebody who is new and familiar, we instantly put him or her in one or more categories. These categories are linked in our minds with specific beliefs that tell us what members of that category are like. For example, the category of "women" is often associated in our minds with adjectives such as warm, nurturing, and yielding, and the category of "men" is often associated with qualities such as assertiveness, decisiveness, and influence. This pattern explains why men are more likely to be chosen as leaders in all kinds of situations. The qualities that we associate with good leadership are more strongly associated with men than women. When it comes time to choose an individual for a leadership position, these strong associations tend to bias us against selecting a woman, even if we consciously believe that men and women are equally good at leadership.

Where do our biases come from? Psychologists believe that we learn them, starting at an early age, from our family, friends, teachers, and the media. There is evidence that young children often hold the same biases that adults do. For example, when asked to draw a scientist, the majority of elementary school students draw a Caucasian-American man in a white lab coat. Since unconscious bias originates from the society in which we live, most of us tend to hold similar biases, regardless of who we are. Men and women are both likely to hold a bias that women are less effective leaders than men. When asked to draw a scientist, even African-American children are more likely to draw a Caucasian-American scientist.

Research has found that our unconscious biases tend to be stable over time. They are so ingrained in us that at the fundamental level they are probably exceedingly difficult to change. However, by becoming more aware of them, we may be able to self-correct for their influence on our behavior.

Measuring Unconscious Bias

How can we know our unconscious biases? Psychologists have developed a computer-based test, called the Implicit Association Test (IAT) that can detect the type and strength of people's unconscious biases. The IAT does this by measuring the speed at which we associate a set of words or images with one category or another. For example, in an IAT assessing unconscious race bias, respondents are asked to quickly classify African-American or Caucasian-American sounding names with the categories "good" or "bad." The speed with which a respondent pairs good or bad words with either race represents his or her unconscious bias. The IAT has been found to be robust at detecting many different types of bias (e.g., race, gender, social class) and has become a widely used research tool. A number of studies suggest that the IAT has the ability to predict future behavior. For example, scores have been used to predict how close someone who is White will choose to sit next to someone who is Black and the likelihood that a woman will pursue a high-status career.

The Effects of Unconscious Bias

In the context of academic medicine, women and minority faculty may be especially vulnerable to the effects of unconscious bias. Although most people express a conscious desire to be fair and objective, unconscious bias influences the way they perceive other people. One study found that employers preferred job candidates with Caucasian names to those with African-American names, even though the study was set up so that all the resumes were identical in their qualifications. A similar study found that male and female psychology professors preferred to hire a male candidate over a female candidate for a faculty position in psychology, even though both candidates had identical curriculum vitae.

Women and minority medical school faculty are at special risk because of long-standing stereotypes that question their scientific and intellectual abilities. In addition to contributing to discrimination, these stereotypes can also undermine the performance of women and minorities through the phenomenon of *stereotype threat*. Introduced by social psychologist Claude Steele in 1995, stereotype threat describes the fear or anxiety that individuals face in situations where they might confirm a negative stereotype about their social group. This anxiety does not need to be conscious in order to disrupt intellectual performance, nor do individuals need to personally endorse the stereotype in order to suffer from its ill effects.

Stereotype threat happens because of the shared knowledge that people have about the stereotypes that exist about certain groups of people. The mere threat of confirming the negative stereotype is enough to disrupt people's actual performance. Studies have shown that women perform worse on math tests after being reminded of the stereotype that women lack mathematical ability. Similarly, African-American students perform worse on the SAT after being told that the test is a valid measure of intelligence. Fortunately, social scientists have begun to develop interventions that can prevent stereotype threat from happening. We turn to these and other strategies below.

Addressing Unconscious Bias

Our underlying unconscious biases are difficult to change. However, there is promising new evidence that we can take steps to consciously self-correct for them, thereby limiting their influence on our thoughts and behavior. Here are several suggestions for a faculty member on how to counter the effects of unconscious bias in academic medicine.

Promote Awareness in Self and Others

By reading this chapter, the academic physician has already begun the first step: becoming more aware of what unconscious bias is and how it affects people's behaviors. It is also important to educate others about unconscious bias. When the issue of stereotyping occurs in conversation, it helps to be knowledgeable about findings that show how unconscious bias can affect important decisions. The physician may want to take the Implicit Association Test (available online), as it can be a useful experience for learning about one's biases. Sharing one's own biases can help others feel more secure about exploring their own. To protect against the influence of unconscious bias on one's judgments about other people, one must pay close attention to the specific thoughts that may be driving one's opinions about others. In addition, being open to alternate perspectives and opposing viewpoints may help the physician become more aware of the unconscious biases that drive his or her and others' opinions.

There is growing evidence that the widespread education of faculty members about unconscious bias may help remove barriers that prevent underrepresented groups from succeeding. The University of Wisconsin developed several hiring workshops for faculty that included information on unconscious bias and how it affects decision making. Those departments where faculty members participated in the workshops showed significantly higher odds of increasing their percentages of women faculty than departments where no one participated.

There is also evidence that teaching people about the cause and consequences of stereotype threat can help them avoid its detrimental influence. One study found that teaching women about stereotype threat and its potential effects on math performance caused their scores on a math test to increase. The implication of this finding, as the title of that study suggests, is that "knowing is half the battle." If other members of his or her department are open to it, the academic physician may want to lead a discussion on unconscious bias. If one does bring up unconscious bias with one's colleagues, one would do well to emphasize that the potential effects apply to everyone. It is not a matter of just some people holding prejudices—we all are vulnerable to letting our biases influence our judgments.

Adopting a "Growth" Mindset

What do academic physicians do when they suspect they may be on the receiving end of unconscious bias? Recognizing that the work climate may not be entirely fair can be very threatening. Indeed, there is evidence that many people would rather blame themselves than accept the possibility that the system may be unfair. When people perceive their environment as unfair, they start to feel helpless and unmotivated. Research on how people respond and cope with failure suggests that a person can cope better with a difficult environment by adopting the right mindset. Specifically, adopting a "growth" mindset may buffer people against the negative effects of being stereotyped. Carol Dweck, a developmental psychologist, has conducted a number of studies revealing how having either a "fixed" or "growth" mindset powerfully affects our potential for future success.

People with a fixed mindset tend to view human abilities, such as intelligence, as stable and difficult to change. In contrast, people with a growth mindset view human abilities as malleable and changeable through sustained effort. Fixed versus growth beliefs about intelligence have important implications for how well people do at school and in their careers. People who believe that intelligence is fixed from birth tend to experience more distress and give up more easily when faced with challenges. Meanwhile, people with growth mindsets tend to bounce back quickly from setbacks and persist longer in the face of difficulty.

These differences in mindset have particular relevance to people who belong to stereotyped groups. Because people with fixed mindsets view human traits as inherent and stable, they are more prone towards stereotyping others. They are also less likely to cope well in environments where stereotypes are pervasive. For example, in her study of women in a high-level calculus course, Dweck found that only those women with fixed mindsets seemed to react badly to the perceived stereotype that women are less gifted at math. By the end of the course, many of them no longer intended to pursue math in the future. In another study, researchers found that African-American students who had a fixed mindset were less likely to incorporate constructive criticism about their intellectual work, whereas students with growth mindsets were less likely to become discouraged after setbacks and more likely to view difficult situations as challenges rather than threats. Adopting a growth mindset is helpful for many people, but it might be especially important for individuals who belong to negatively stereotyped groups.

How does one develop a growth mindset? Although it may seem difficult to change, Dweck has been able to change people's mindsets in experimental settings. Dweck suggests the following steps:

1. *Pay attention to what you are telling yourself.* When you succeed, do you think it is because of your natural ability or because of the effort you put out? Do you see failures as indicative of your inherent ability?

2. *Recognize that you have a choice.* It is possible to interpret failure in different ways. It is possible to view a rejection or a setback as a challenge rather than a disaster.

3. *Talk back to your fixed mindset "voice."* Instead of telling yourself that your manuscript being rejected is proof that you shouldn't pursue an academic career, remind yourself that it is an opportunity to improve your work and your knowledge of how to publish successfully.

4. *Accept challenges and interpret the results within a growth mindset.* Often when we have a fixed mindset, we avoid doing things that seem risky. By making it okay for yourself to fail, you can take on new challenges without too much fear and anxiety. If you do fail, interpret it as a learning experience and nothing more.

Expanding Networks

In addition to focusing one's mindset, connecting with others and expanding one's professional networks can also be helpful in countering the effects of unconscious bias. Stereotypes can lower one's sense of belonging to an environment, which may have discouraging effects on one's career. Research shows, for instance, that women who do not feel that they belong in computer science are less likely to pursue careers in it, even when they have high aptitudes. Individuals who belong to stereotyped groups are at greater risk of feeling isolated, especially in mainstream institutions like school and work. Uncertainty about belonging can undermine performance and well-being and pose significant challenges to career development and advancement.

Developing connections to colleagues and similar others not only provides an important source of professional support but also serves as a buffer against the effects that a low sense of belonging can have on actual performance. Networks provide many positive effects, such as mentoring, access to information and opportunities, and professional and personal support. Specific to unconscious bias, connecting with others can also increase your sense of belonging, thereby protecting against feelings of isolation that may accompany stereotype threat. Recent experimental research shows that interventions, such as learning that others have faced similar adversities, can increase one's sense of belonging and thereby elevate one's well-being and performance. Building one's networks allows for exchange and sharing of experiences, which can alleviate the doubt and uncertainty that stereotypes can create.

Professional Development

Being proactive in one's career advancement process can be critical to overcoming unconscious bias. Below are some specific strategies that faculty members can consider using:

1. *Communicate with supervisors.* It is easy to assume that your unit head or other evaluators already know everything there is to know about you. However, studies on hiring and promotion show that evaluators tend to fall back on stereotypes when they have missing, incomplete, or ambiguous information. It is important to make sure that your evaluators are fully aware of your background and qualifications. For example, when requesting a letter of recommendation, provide your recommender with detailed information about your background and qualifications.
2. *Critically examine the resources allocated to you.* Unconscious bias often manifests itself in the amount of resources allocated to members of one group versus another. Do you feel you have the resources you need to accomplish your research and other work activities? If your resources seem scant, especially compared to your colleagues, actively seek out ways to get more of what you need. Differences in resources might seem small on the surface, but over time they can significantly affect how successful you are in the long-run.
3. *Do not be afraid to self-nominate.* When the NIH Pioneer Awards began to allow for self-nominations, the number of women nominees and recipients increased dramatically. People may unintentionally overlook certain people for awards because of unconscious bias. Therefore, you should not be afraid of nominating yourself for awards and other opportunities.

Institutional Recommendations

Although we have outlined a number of recommendations in this chapter that individuals can act upon, a long-term strategy for combatting the effects of unconscious bias on faculty careers must include institutional commitment. Actions taken at the institutional level can go a long way in reducing the impact of unconscious bias on hiring and promotion. In addition to educating organizational leaders on unconscious bias, institutions can create ground rules for hiring and promotion to ensure equity in the employment process. For example, it is important to assign someone or appoint a committee with the role of overseeing hiring practices. Such oversight may include paying attention to the language in job postings and flyers and encouraging the active recruitment of candidates from underrepresented groups. Another important strategy for institutions is to require sufficient diversity among search committees. A study on law firms revealed that the odds of a female hire increases when women are included in the evaluative and decision-making process (e.g., as a hiring partner). In addition, setting criteria before evaluating candidates can ensure that criteria do not shift to fit the favored candidate. Creating a key set of questions for the interview can ensure that discussions about the candidates focus on job-related factors.

Words to the Wise
- Mental shortcuts become a problem when they lead to stereotyping.
- By becoming more aware of unconscious biases, we may be able to self-correct for their influence on our behavior.
- Networks provide many positive effects, such as mentoring, access to information and opportunities, and professional and personal support.

Ask Your Mentor or Colleagues
- How aware are people at this institution about unconscious bias and the potential role it plays in faculty careers?
- Does the institution have any programs, initiatives, or guidelines that may help in combatting unconscious bias? If no, what might be a way to develop some?
- Are there other faculty, with backgrounds similar to my own, to whom you could introduce me?
- Are there career development, mentoring, or professional networking programs at this institution in which you would recommend that I participate?

Further Reading

Aboud FE. The development of prejudice in childhood and adolescence. In: Dovidio JF, Glick P, Rudman LA, editors. On the nature of prejudice. Malden, MA: Blackwell; 2005. p. 310–26.

Amodio DM. Devine PG Stereotyping and evaluation in implicit race bias: evidence for independent constructs and unique effects on behavior. J Pers Soc Psychol. 2006;91:652–61.

Aronson J, Fried CB, Good C. Reducing the effects of stereotype threat on African-American college students by shaping theories of intelligence. J Exp Soc Psychol. 2002;38:113–25.

Association of American Medical Colleges. 2011 applicant enrollment data. https://www.aamc.org/download/264082/data/applicantenrollment-data2011.pdf. Accessed 14 Feb 2012.

Association of American Medical Colleges. The changing demographics of full-time U.S. medical school faculty, 1966–2009. https://www.aamc.org/download/266758/data/aibvol11_no8.pdf. Accessed 13 Feb 2012.

Association of American Medical Colleges. Women in academic medicine statistics and medical school benchmarking, 2009–2010. https://www.aamc.org/members/gwims/statistics/. Accessed 13 Feb 2012.

Association of American Medical Colleges. Unconscious bias in faculty and leadership recruitment: a literature review. https://www.aamc.org/download/102364/data/aibvol9no2.pdf. Accessed 24 Feb 2012.

Bertrand M, Mullainathan S. Are Emily and Greg more employable than Lakisha and Jamal? A field experiment on labor market discrimination. Am Econ Rev. 2004;94:991–1013.

Blackwell LS, Trzesniewski KH, Dweck CS. Implicit theories of intelligence predict achievement across an adolescent transition: a longitudinal study and an intervention. Child Dev. 2007;78:246–63.

Bragger JD, Kutcher E, Morgan J, Firth P. The effects of the structured interview on reducing biases against pregnant job applicants. Sex Roles. 2002;46:215–26.

Carnes M. Gender: macho language and other deterrents. Nature. 2006; 442:868.

Cheryan S, Plaut G, Davies PG, Steele CM. Ambient belonging: how stereotypical cues impact gender participation in computer science. J Pers Soc Psychol. 2009;97:1045–60.

Croskerry P. A universal model of diagnostic reasoning. Acad Med. 2009;84:1022–8.

Eagly AH, Karau SJ. Role congruity theory of prejudice toward female leaders. Psychol Rev. 2002;109:573–98.

Dweck CS. Self-theories: their role in motivation, personality, and development. Philadelphia: Psychology Press; 1999.

Dweck CS. Mindset: the new psychology of success. New York: Random House; 2006a.

Dweck CS. Is math a gift? Beliefs that put females at risk. In: Ceci SJ, Williams W, editors. Why aren't more women in science? Top researchers debate the evidence. Washington, DC: American Psychological Association; 2006b.

Finson KD. Drawing a scientist: what we do and do not know after fifty years of drawings. Sch Sci Math. 2002;102:335–45.

Fiske ST. Social cognition and the normality of prejudgment. In: Dovidio JF, Glick P, Rudman LA, editors. On the nature of prejudice. Malden, MA: Blackwell; 2005. p. 36–53.

Greenwald AG, Banaji MR. Implicit social cognition: attitudes, self-esteem, and stereotypes. Psychol Rev. 1995;102:4–27.

Greenwald AG, McGhee DE, Schwartz JLK. Measuring individual differences in implicit cognition: the implicit association test. J Pers Soc Psychol. 1998;74:1464–80.

Greenwald AG, Poehlman TA, Uhlmann EL, Banaji MR. Understanding and using the implicit association test, III: meta-analysis of predictive validity. J Pers Soc Psychol. 2009;97:17–41.

Gorman E. Gender stereotypes, same-gender preferences, and organizational variation in the hiring of women: evidence from law firms. Am Sociol Rev. 2005;70:702–28.

Gorman E. Work uncertainty and the promotion of professional women: the case of law firm partnership. Soc Forces. 2006;85:865–90.

Heilman ME, Block CJ, Stathatos P. The affirmative action stigma of incompetence: effects of performance information ambiguity. Acad Manage J. 1997;40:603–25.

Heilman ME. Description and prescription: how gender stereotypes prevent women's ascent up the organizational ladder. J Soc Issues. 2001;57: 657–74.

Hitchcock MA, Bland CJ, Hekelman FP, Blumenthal MG. Professional networks: the influence of colleagues on the academic success of faculty. Acad Med. 1995;70:1108–16.

Ito TA, Urland GR. Race and gender on the brain: electrocortical measures of attention to the race and gender of multiply categorizable individuals. J Pers Soc Psychol. 2003;85:616–26.

Johns M, Schmader T, Martens A. Knowing is half the battle: teaching stereotype threat as a means of improving women's math performance. Psychol Sci. 2005;16:175–9.

Jost JT, Rudman LA, Blair IV, Carney DR, Dasgupta N, Glaser J, Hardin CD. The existence of implicit bias is beyond reasonable doubt: a refutation of ideological and methodological objections and executive summary of ten studies that no manager should ignore. Res Organ Behav. 2009;29:39–69.

Kaiser CR, Miller CT. Stop complaining! The social costs of making attributions to discrimination. Pers Soc Psychol Bull. 2001;27:254–63.

Kiefer AK, Sekaquaptewa D. Implicit stereotypes and women's math performance: how implicit gender-math stereotypes influence women's susceptibility to stereotype threat. J Exp Soc Psychol. 2007;43:825–32.

Koenig AM, Eagly AH, Mitchell AA, Ristikari T. Are leader stereotypes masculine? A meta-analysis of three research paradigms. Psychol Bull. 2011;137:616–42.

Lenton AP, Bruder M, Sedikides C. A meta-analysis on the malleability of automatic gender stereotypes. Psychol Women Q. 2009;33:183–96.

Levy S, Stroessner S, Dweck CS. Stereotype formation and endorsement: the role of implicit theories. J Pers Soc Psychol. 1998;74:1421–36.

Lyubormirsky S, Sheldon KM, Schkade D. Pursuing happiness: the architecture of sustainable change. Rev Gen Psychol. 2005;9:111–31.

Massachusetts Institute of Technology. A study on the status of women faculty in science at MIT. http://web.mit.edu/fnl/women/women.html. Accessed 27 Feb 2012.

National Academy of Sciences, National Academy of Engineering, & Institute of Medicine. Beyond bias and barriers: fulfilling the potential of women in academic science and engineering. Washington, DC: National Academies; 2007.

Nosek BA, Banaji MR, Greenwald AG. Harvesting implicit group attitudes and beliefs from a demonstration website. Group Dyn. 2002;6:101–15.

Nosek BA, Greenwald AG, Banaji MR. The implicit association test at age 7: a methodological and conceptual review. In: Bargh J, editor. Automatic processes in social thinking and behavior. London, England: Psychology Press; 2007. p. 265–92.

Project Implicit. https://implicit.harvard.edu/implicit/. Accessed 14 Feb 2012.

Ridgeway CL, Correll SJ. Unpacking the gender system: a theoretical perspective on gender beliefs and social relations. Gend Soc. 2004;18:510–31.

Rudman LA, Glick P. Prescriptive gender stereotypes and backlash toward agentic women. J Soc Issues. 2001;57:743–62.

Rudman LA, Heppen JB. Implicit romantic fantasies and women's interest in personal power: a glass slipper effect? Pers Soc Psychol Bull. 2003;29: 1357–70.

Rudman LA, Fairchild K. Reactions to counterstereotypic behavior: the role of backlash in cultural stereotype maintenance. J Pers Soc Psychol. 2004;87:157–76.

Schmader T, Major B, Gramzow RH. Coping with ethnic stereotypes in the academic domain: perceived injustice and psychological disengagement. J Soc Issues. 2001;57:83–111.

Sheridan JT, Fine E, Pribbenow CM, Handelsman J, Carnes M. Searching for excellence and diversity: increasing the hiring of women faculty at one academic medical center. Acad Med. 2010;85:999–1007.

Steele CM. A threat in the air: how stereotypes shape intellectual identity and performance. Am Psychol. 1997;52:613–29.

Steinpres RE, Anders KA, Ritzke D. The impact of gender on the review of the curricula vitae of job applicants and tenure candidates: a national empirical study. Sex Roles. 2003;41:499–28.

Stewart TL, Latu IM, Kawakami K, Myers AC. Consider the situation: reducing automatic stereotyping through situational attribution training. J Exp Soc Psychol. 2010;46:221–5.

Uhlmann EL, Cohen G. Constructed criteria. Psychol Sci. 2005;16:474–80.

Walton GM, Cohen GL. A question of belonging: race, social fit, and achievement. J Pers Soc Psychol. 2007;92:82–96.

Walton GM, Cohen GL. A brief social-belonging intervention improves academic and health outcomes of minority students. Science. 2011;331: 1147–451.

How to Intervene with Unethical and Unprofessional Colleagues

17

Jerald Belitz

All academic health disciplines have an obligation to delineate their scope of practice, ethical and professional principles, and responsibilities to their patients and communities. Each discipline endeavors to ensure that professionals apply safe and effective interventions to patients, ethically conduct research, and respectfully interact with colleagues and students. As part of this obligation, each profession is expected to develop mechanisms to monitor and regulate the performance of its members.

Accompanying the privilege of self-governance is the responsibility to assertively intercede when an associate evidences unsafe, incompetent, unethical, unprofessional, or illegal behaviors. This ethical responsibility is codified by the American Medical Association [1] and the American Psychological Association [2]. Interventions with unethical peers can range from an informal discussion to a formal report to the State Licensing Board. Interventions protect existing and future patients and maintain the integrity of the profession and affiliated institution. Further, they adhere to the ethical keystones of beneficence, nonmaleficence, integrity, and respect for other's rights and dignity. Several studies [3–7] have conclusively

J. Belitz, Ph.D. (✉)
Department of Psychiatry, University of New Mexico,
2600 Marble NE, Albuquerque, NM, USA
e-mail: Jbelitz@salud.unm.edu

© Springer International Publishing Switzerland 2016
L.W. Roberts (ed.), *The Associate Professor Guidebook*,
DOI 10.1007/978-3-319-28001-1_17

demonstrated that physicians and psychologists, both in training and independent practice, recognize when a colleague violates ethical and professional standards. Yet, the same research reveals a hesitancy or unwillingness to interpose when that colleague displays unacceptable practices.

This chapter will clarify the gradients of unethical and unprofessional behaviors, the aversion of professionals to intercede with errant colleagues, proposed interventions, and recommendations for the prevention of ethical misconduct.

The Spectrum of Ethical Infractions

AMA [1, 8] identifies three substrates for ethical and professional violations: impairment, incompetence, and unethical conduct. Physician impairment is defined as the inability to practice medicine due to physical or mental illness, including deterioration through the aging process, the loss of motor skills, or the excessive use or abuse of drugs, including alcohol. AMA typically focuses on the risk to patients; however, it readily extends to the domains of education and research. Extreme fatigue and emotional stress are subsumed under the rubric of impairment. Interestingly, APA [9] defines emotional stress or distress as an experience of intense stress that affects well-being and functioning or disruption of thinking, mood, and other health problems that interfere with professional functioning. It is depicted as a source of ethical misconduct distinct from impairment. APA defines an impaired psychologist as one who has a condition that may cause harm to the patient or others. From this stage forward, the term *impairment* will incorporate the construct of distress.

Levels of physical and psychological impairment among health-care professionals are congruent with the rates in the general population. For example, approximately 15 % of medical professionals will experience problems with alcohol and/or substance abuse at some point in their career [10, 11]. However, physicians are twice as likely as the general public to complete suicide [12–14]. Extreme stress related to health-care work has been identified as one of the causes of depression and substance abuse [15].

As a result of their recurring exposure to patients with enduring medical, physical, and emotional difficulties, health-care professionals are more disposed to distress and, in its extreme manifestation, burnout [9, 12, 16]. More specifically, providers can experience stress as a result of containing their own emotional response to others' pain; maintaining therapeutic boundaries; negotiating competing demands from patients, medical institutions, insurance companies, and regulatory entities; balancing their clinical and academic responsibilities; and confronting their imperfections as clinicians or teachers.

Incompetence refers to the provision of substandard levels of patient care due to inadequate knowledge, skills, or judgment [1, 8]. Again this can be translated to include deficiencies in the areas of education and research. Incompetent care is often difficult to discern because one customarily needs to observe a pattern of errors or poor outcomes before concluding the colleague is practicing at a substandard level. Morreim [17] cautions against equating adverse treatment outcomes with incompetent care. Poor outcomes may also result from natural factors beyond human control, unexpected effects despite a well-justified intervention, atypical but not necessarily unacceptable interventions, or good management of a remarkably complex circumstance.

Though impaired and incompetent providers evidence unethical activities, AMA [1, 8] characterizes unethical conduct as an array of infractions that involves exploitation of patients, colleagues, or students; boundary violations; fraud; dishonesty; greed; and violations of professional guidelines. Academic medical institutions also require principled behavior and adherence to ethical and legal guidelines among their professionals. As an illustration, the University of New Mexico [18] has a policy that identifies additional examples of misconduct including discrimination, sexual harassment, willful failure to perform duties, unauthorized release of confidential information, falsification of documents or reports, and any retaliation against an employee who reports misconduct. Essentially, through their behavior, these professionals place their own needs above those of others. In some situations practitioners may be unaware of specific codes of ethics. In other cases, clinicians disregard ethical and professional standards in a manipulative and deliberate effort to gratify their own interests.

Culture of Silence

It is well established that mental health professionals have the awareness of professional ethics and the acumen to identify unethical practices; however, a significant number of clinicians remain uncomfortable and reluctant to report or intervene with their unprincipled colleagues. A recent study [5] revealed that more than one-third of physicians did not fully endorse the ethical tenet that impaired or incompetent colleagues should be reported to a licensing or credentialing board. Historically, this refusal has been branded as a "code of silence" or "culture of silence" or "conspiracy of silence" [11, 19–21]. Multiple personal, interpersonal, and contextual factors account for this silence.

After the fact of discovering that a colleague has been unethical, several clinicians struggle with the dilemma of either protecting the privacy and confidentiality of their colleague or securing the safety and well-being of the patient, student, research subject, or public. Those who honor their societal obligations over the individual rights of the offending colleague are more likely to report the unethical behavior [6]. Others choose to not act because they are apprehensive that a report will cause their colleague to be, for example, stigmatized as an alcoholic, drug addict, mentally ill, deviant, or any other iteration of unfit; unfairly punished; or disallowed to practice his or her chosen profession. It is assumed a report will engender financial difficulties, marital and family problems, humiliation, depression, and further emotional deterioration for their coworker. Others use rationalization, believing their colleague will "work it out" or expecting the problem to disappear [11]. And still others avoid the distress that comes with confronting a colleague. Many identify with their errant colleague, agonizing that they too could have a lapse of moral reasoning and believing they deserve a second chance to right their mistakes and confirm they are ethical professionals.

A fear of retribution from the reported party, peers, supervisors, or the medical institution itself inhibits professionals from acting ethically. Despite the specific language and protection from codes of ethics and university policies, the reporting provider may worry about a subsequent lawsuit for slander, libel, or discrimination [17].

The reporting provider may be identified as a whistle-blower [17] and subsequently endure a loss of status from peers, supervisors, or administrators. Negative consequences could include a sense of isolation among peers, an inability to advance one's career through promotions or new professional opportunities, or a decline in referrals and a loss of income. Not surprisingly, power differentials often preclude trainees and professionals from reporting or intervening when they observe unethical or incompetent behavior by a section chief, chair, or any other person in a position of sanctioned authority.

Reasons to Intervene

Simply stated, there are three fundamental reasons for intervening with an impaired, incompetent, or unethical colleague: prevention of harm to patients or others, prevention of harm to one's profession, and assistance to impaired peers.

Ethical interventions protect existing and future patients. Beneficence and nonmaleficence, the duty to act for the benefit of the patient and, in the least, to do no harm, are the core principles of the Hippocratic Oath [12]. Subsequent to the Hippocratic Oath, health professions have cultivated ethics codes that guide conduct in the spheres of patient care, self-care, education, research, hospital relations, interprofessional relations, and social policy. Professionals are not only directed to monitor their own behaviors but also to intercede on behalf of patients or others when a colleague violates professional standards.

Health professions are allowed significant autonomy to define and regulate themselves through the process of selecting whom to train, developing the training curriculum, defining practice standards, licensing practitioners, and disciplining members [22, 23]. Academic institutions, via the accreditation methodology, coordinate with these professional associations to ensure that trainees are prepared to competently and ethically practice in their specific fields. It is reasoned that only these professionals have the unique knowledge and expertise to execute self-regulation in the endeavor to promote and protect the welfare of the community. Failure to self-govern generates mistrust in the professions and their affiliated associations and institutions. Inadequate interventions with unethical or incompetent colleagues will inexorably lead to increased control by external government and regulatory entities, resulting in the diminishment of professional autonomy. These intrusions may adversely affect the patient–provider relationship, the educator–learner relationship, and other academic pursuits.

Medical associations in all 50 states have initiated impaired physician programs [8]. Likewise, other professional societies and state licensing boards have colleague assistance programs. This nonpunitive approach to treatment and rehabilitation has proven to be effective in reinstating impaired professionals to safe practices. Physician recovery rates from substance abuse are higher than the general population [11] and are estimated to be 78 % [24]. The evidence indicates that interventions which provide structure and strict monitoring are the most effective [25]. These programs allow for patients to have access to a greater number of providers; protect society's investment in training highly skilled providers, scientists, and educators; and demonstrate the profession's commitment to monitoring its members.

Interventions

All academic institutions and Health Sciences Centers have policies delineating unprofessional, unethical, and illegal behaviors and procedures for intervening with or reporting errant colleagues. UNM will again serve as a representative example. UNM's policy manuals [18, 26] encompass measures for patient care and safety, sexual harassment, discrimination, research fraud, conflicts of interest, misconduct, and protections for whistle-blowers. Reporting procedures include communication with supervisors and relevant university compliance offices such as the Division of Human Resources, Office of Equal Opportunity, Research Compliance Services, and Offices of Clinical Affairs or Academic Affairs. UNM also has a dispute resolution service that provides consultation and mediation services to faculty and administrators for workplace conflicts or for grievances regarding violations of UNM policies and practices. Faculty members are educated about these policies during their initial orientation and are required to pass annual on-line competencies to ensure their ongoing knowledge and adherence.

Professional associations have codes of ethics and conduct. AMA [1, 8] has guidelines for confronting its three forms of unethical behavior. A nonpunitive approach is used with substandard colleagues. With regard to impaired colleagues, professionals are expected to communicate with them in an effort to have that colleague discontinue practice and enroll in a sanctioned physician assistance program. Clearly, this information must be shared with that individual's department chair and the institution's oversight committees. A report to the state licensing board is mandated if the colleague continues to practice or resumes practice without concordance from the assistance program.

Incompetent physicians are initially reported to the appropriate service chief or administrator who has the authority to assess the potential impact on the patients' welfare and to facilitate remedial action for the errant provider. This authorized individual is obliged to notify the hospital peer review entity and ensure that the identified deficiencies are remedied. When the incompetence represents immediate threat to the patient, that patient must be immediately protected, and a report must be made directly to the state licensing board. If the incompetent physician fails to access or benefit from remediation, a report is also made to the licensing board.

Other unethical behaviors are reported to the appropriate service supervisor. If the unethical behavior continues, further reports are made to individuals or offices with increasing amounts of authority to evaluate and discipline the offending physician. Reports are always sent to the state licensing board and/or law enforcement agencies when the misconduct violates licensing standards or criminal laws.

An ethics primer prepared by one medical specialty society [23] proposes a four-step ethical decision-making process to help determine the best course of action with unethical colleagues:

1. Be aware of your state's reporting requirements as specified by legal statutes and licensing boards (and also the university and hospital policies). Become knowledgeable about local resources available to assist impaired or naive peers.

2. Evaluate the source of information, confirm the information, and determine the nature of the violations with regard to ethical and professional standards. Attend to any personal values or emotions that are triggered by the information.
3. Identify potential interventions and possible competing interests in each option. Identify personal reactions to the various options.
4. Select the most appropriate option, knowing other options are available. Other options may be used as needed. Preserve the goal of protecting patients and maintaining the highest professional standards.

Implicit in these suggestions and in all other ethical guidelines is the reminder to consult with a peer who is aware of ethical and legal practices and is willing to provide honest, unadorned, and meaningful feedback.

The Ethical Principles of Psychologists and Code of Conduct [2] demarcates formal and informal actions that are available to professionals who observe colleague misconduct. This approach is a useful model for other health professions as well. Although a referral to a colleague assistance program is endorsed, it is not required by the ethics code or accepted as a substitute for a formal or informal action. For ethical violations that have not caused substantial harm to a patient or others, psychologists are encouraged to informally resolve the concern via a discussion with the errant colleague. Substantial harm is not specifically defined, compelling the practitioner to determine if an informal intervention is indicated. Examples of observed breaches that may prompt an informal approach include recurrent lateness for patient appointments, leaving medical records unconcealed overnight, or a discussion among colleagues about patients in an inappropriate environment even if it appears nobody can eavesdrop. Of course nonclinical violations, such as argumentative and rude interactions with colleagues, can also be addressed with an informal intervention.

Optimally, this procedure is conducted in a nonadversarial, constructive, and educational manner. However, this process can be uncomfortable and even perceived as a confrontation. Several important ethicists [27–30] have outlined guidelines for an interpersonal intervention with an unethical colleague. A synthesis of their work allows for the following recommendations. These recommendations are appropriate whenever a professional challenges a colleague's ability to perform his or her responsibilities safely and ethically.

1. Collect information about the offending behavior and determine the strength and veracity of the evidence. Evaluate it within the context of the relevant sections of the Code of Ethics and Conduct.
2. Explore one's motivation to engage in or avoid this process. The primary motivation needs to be the welfare of the injured party.
3. Consult with a trusted colleague who has experience and knowledge of professionalism and ethics. This colleague is trusted to evaluate the information in an unbiased and informed manner, irrespective of one's personal relationship with the consultant.
4. Determine who will talk to the errant colleague. This is likely to be the individual who observed the misconduct. If an imbalance of power exists, it may be judicious to have a professional of equal power employ this role. The imbalance of power can encompass differentials in assigned roles and authority, gender, or ethnicity.
5. Maintain an educational and emotionally neutral demeanor without reacting to any negative affect by the refractory colleague. Listen to the colleague's perspective and reasoning for the inappropriate behavior; ask for additional information and clarification.
6. Structure the intervention with the aim of jointly identifying goals and objectives, useful resources, an action plan, and a follow-up plan.

APA cautions that the confidentiality of an injured patient must not be compromised in this process.

APA requires a more aggressive endeavor if the unethical behavior causes or is liable to cause substantial harm or if an informal action has not produced an adequate resolution. This involves protecting patients or others from imminent harm. A formal report is made to a state or national ethics committee, licensing board, and/or institutional oversight committee.

Recommendations

Historically professionalism and ethics were learned indirectly through lectures or observing supervisors [31, 32]. Medical students and residents encountered poor role modeling and witnessed ethical dilemmas being ignored or unresolved. Further, these trainees were not taught the importance of self-care. Instead, they learned to not seek assistance for health problems for fear of academic reprisals [33]. Consequently, professionals' attitudes and practices concerning ethics are frequently the ones they encountered in their training. In a significant effort to remedy this state of affairs, the Accreditation Council for Graduate Medical Education directed medical schools to include professionalism as a core competency by the year 2007. There is evidence that this effort is yielding positive results; physicians in practice less than 10 years are more likely to report a refractory colleague than physicians with more than 10 years of practice [5]. It can be expected that future providers will be better equipped to perform their ethical responsibilities and negotiate the internal and external conflicts associated with inappropriate colleagues.

Additional education is essential for more senior providers. Professional societies, licensing boards, and credentialing committees are in excellent positions to mandate and offer professionalism and ethics in-service training as a requisite for certification or licensing. Credentialing committees can also institute peer review processes that assess ethical functioning. As the professions move towards a treatment and educational model, intercessions reduce the stigma and risks for both the reporting and imprudent practitioners.

Both the AMA and the APA have ethical guidelines charging providers to obtain suitable help if they experience a personal, medical, psychological, or stress-related condition. It is crucial for professionals to maintain a state of wellness and health so that they can proficiently perform their responsibilities without submitting to the strain of managing the multiple roles and tasks associated with a medical academic career. Providers are expected to engage in self-care, ongoing professional development, and consultation with trusted colleague. A well lived and balanced life is the best antidote to stress and carelessness.

Reasons to Intervene

- Safety and well-being of patients and society.
- Integrity and autonomy of one's profession.
- Assistance for impaired peers.

Words to the Wise
- Reasons to intervene include safety and well-being of patients and society; integrity and autonomy of one's profession; and assistance for impaired peers.
- Collect information and evaluate it within the context of legal and ethics standards.
- Explore one's motivation. The primary motivation is the welfare of the injured party.
- Consult with a colleague who has experience and knowledge of professionalism and ethics.
- Determine who will talk to the errant colleague.
- Maintain an educational and emotionally neutral demeanor.
- Identify goals and objectives, useful resources, an action plan, and a follow-up plan.

Ask Your Mentor or Colleagues
- How can I determine if a colleague is impaired?
- What should I do if I observe my supervisor engaging in incompetent behavior?
- Am I obligated to intervene when I see a respected colleague evidence unethical behavior?
- Under what circumstances am I obligated to report errant behavior to a licensing or credentialing board?
- What can I do to ensure that I maintain ethical and competent practices?

References

1. Council on Ethical and Judicial Affairs. Code of medical ethics of the American Medical Association (2008–2009 edition). Chicago: American Medical Association; 2008.
2. American Psychological Association. Ethical principles of psychologists and code of conduct: 2010 amendments. 2010. http://www.apa.org/ethics/code/index.aspx. Accessed 19 Dec 2011.
3. Bernard JL, Jara CS. The failure of clinical psychology graduate students to apply understood ethical principles. Prof Psychol Res Pract. 1986;17:313–5.
4. Bernard JL, Murphy M, Little M. The failure of clinical psychologists to apply understood ethical principles. Prof Psychol Res Pract. 1987;18:489–91.
5. DesRoches CM, Rao SR, Fromson JA, et al. Physician's perceptions, preparedness for reporting, and experience related to impaired and incompetent colleagues. J Am Med Assoc. 2010;304:187–93.
6. Farber NJ, Gilbert SG, Aboff BM, et al. Physician's willingness to report impaired colleagues. Soc Sci Med. 2005;61:1772–5.
7. Wilkins MA, McGuire JM, Abbott DW, Blau BI. Willingness to apply understood ethical principles. J Clin Psychol. 1990;46:539–47.
8. Council on Ethical and Judicial Affairs. Reporting impaired, incompetent or unethical colleagues. CEJA Report A – I-91; 1992.
9. American Psychology Association Advisory Committee on Colleague Assistance. The stress–distress-impairment continuum for psychologists. n.d. http://www.apapracticecentral.org/ce/self-care/colleague-assist.aspx. Accessed 16 Dec 2011.
10. Baldisseri MR. Impaired healthcare professional. Crit Care Med 2007;35(Suppl.): S106–16.
11. Boisaubin EV, Levine RE. Identifying and assisting the impaired physician. Am J Med Sci. 2001;322:31–6.
12. Roberts LW, Dyer AR. Ethics in mental health care. Washington, D.C.: American Psychiatric Publishing; 2004.
13. Wilson A, Rosen A, Randal P, et al. Psychiatrically impaired medical practitioners: an overview with special reference to impaired psychiatrists. Australas Psychiatry. 2009;17:6–10.
14. Dhai A, Szabo CP, McQuoid-Mason DJ. The impaired practitioner – scope of the problem and ethical challenges. S Afr Med J. 2006;96:1069–72.
15. Carinci AJ, Christo PJ. Physician impairment: is recovery feasible? Pain Phys J. 2009;12:487–91.
16. Layman MJ, McNamara RJ. Remediation for ethics violations: focus on psychotherapists' sexual contact with clients. Prof Psychol Res Pract. 1997;28:281–92.
17. Morreim EH. Am I my brother's warden? Responding to the unethical or incompetent colleague. Hastings Cent Rep. 1993;23:19–27.

18. University of New Mexico. Board of regents policy manual. 2010. http://www.unm.edu/~brpm/rtoc.htm. Accessed 19 Dec 2011.
19. Cohen S. The conspiracy of silence. Can Fam Phys. 1980;26:847–9.
20. Mustard LW. The culture of silence: disruptive and impaired physicians. J Med Pract Manage. 2009;25:153–5.
21. Pope KS, Tabachnick BG, Keith-Spiegel P. The beliefs and behaviors of psychologists as therapists. Am Psychol. 1987;42:993–1006.
22. Lo B. Resolving ethical dilemmas: a guide for clinicians. 3rd ed. New York: Lippincott Williams & Wilkins; 2005.
23. Overstreet MM. Duty to report colleagues who engage in fraud or deception. In: American Psychiatric Association, editors. Ethics primer of the American Psychiatric Association. Washington, DC: American Psychiatric Association; 2001, p. 51–55.
24. Merlo LJ, Altenburger KM, Gold MS. Physician's experience with impaired colleagues. J Am Med Assoc. 2010;304:1895.
25. Rosen A, Wison A, Randal P, Pethebridge A, Codyre D, Barton D, Norrie P, McGeorge P, Rose L. Psychiatrically impaired medical practitioners: better care to reduce harm and life impact, with special reference to impaired psychiatrists. Australas Psychiatry. 2009;17:11–8.
26. University of New Mexico. University business policies and procedures manual. 2012. http://www.unm.edu/~ubppm/ubppmanual/2200. Accessed 10 Jan 12.
27. Koocher GP, Keith-Spiegel P. Ethics in psychology and the mental health professions: standards and cases. New York: Oxford University Press; 2008.
28. O'Connor MF, APA Advisory Committee on Colleague Assistance. Intervening with an impaired colleague. n.d. http://www.apapracticecentral.org/ce/self-care/intervening.aspx. Accessed 16 Dec 2011.
29. Pope KS, Vasquez MJT. Ethics in psychotherapy and counseling: a practical guide. 3rd ed. San Francisco: Jossey-Bass; 2007.
30. VandenBos GR, Duthie RF. Confronting and supporting colleagues in distress. In: Kilburg R, Nathan P, Thoreson R, editors. Professionals in distress. Washington, DC: American Psychological Association; 1986. p. 211–32.
31. Belitz J. On professionalism. In: Roberts LW, Hoop J, editors. Professionalism and ethics: Q & A self-study guide for mental health professionals. Washington, DC: American Psychiatric Publishing; 2008, p. 73–78.
32. D'eon M, Lear N, Turner M, Jones C. Perils of the hidden curriculum revisited. Med Teach. 2007;29:295–6.
33. Roberts LW, Warner TD, et al. Perceptions of academic vulnerability associated with personal illness: a study of 1,027 students at nine medical schools. Compr Psychiatry. 2001;42:1–15.

How to Participate in Ethics Committees

18

Ryan Spellecy, Cynthiane Morgenweck, and Arthur R. Derse

If you are considering serving on an ethics committee, whether by invitation or your own initiative, it is important that you first understand the role of an ethics committee. Confusion regarding the role of ethics committees, as well as a perception of ineffectiveness of ethics committees, stems from a misunderstanding of the committee's basic purpose. The misunderstanding is that ethics committees "tell people what to do" and usurp the autonomy of the caregiving team. It is erroneous to believe that ethics committees direct patient care and that clinicians are obliged to follow the recommendations of the committee. An ethics committee is not the "ethics police." Indeed, nothing could be further from the truth.

In actual practice, ethics committee consultations are nondirective and strictly advisory. This means that the recommendations they might issue are not binding for the attending physician or anyone else. In that regard, an ethics consultation is similar to other requests for consultation. An attending physician might request a consultation from nephrology but is not required to follow the recommendations from the nephrologist.

Also, ethics committees do much more than ethics consultation. Ethics committees have three functions: education, policy development and review, and consultation [1]. Some have argued that if

R. Spellecy, Ph.D. (✉)
Center for Bioethics and Medical Humanities, Medical College of Wisconsin, 8701 Watertown Plank Road, Milwaukee, WI, USA
e-mail: rspellec@mcw.edu

© Springer International Publishing Switzerland 2016
L.W. Roberts (ed.), *The Associate Professor Guidebook*,
DOI 10.1007/978-3-319-28001-1_18

an ethics committee excels at the first two functions, ethics consultation might actually decrease as staff become better educated regarding how to approach ethical dilemmas. Moreover, when policies at the institution are clear enough to provide sufficient guidance to resolve many dilemmas, there is lessened need for the involvement of the ethics committee. Paradoxically, though, consults may increase as clinicians may become more aware of issues and the help the ethics committee may give, and patients and families may be more comfortable in requesting a consult. The data on this subject simply do not exist, and in our clinical ethics experience, we have seen both cases occur.

So, to return to the initial question, let's assume you are considering serving on an ethics committee. If you are considering this because you see problems at your institution that you believe have an ethical component and your goal is to serve on the ethics committee in order to "fix" those problems, the ethics committee may not be the right fit for you. Ethics committees should neither desire nor have the authority to force people to choose a particular course of action. As one author notes, members of ethics committees should be well respected not only for their clinical judgment but also for their interpersonal skills [2]. So, if you are the type of person in whom colleagues confide and whose judgment is valued when colleagues are wrestling with issues and if you have a passion not for solving problems but for equipping your colleagues with the ethical background to help them resolve problems, participation in an ethics committee can be a meaningful and fruitful mechanism for you to serve your institution and your colleagues.

Composition of an Ethics Committee

Ethics committees are found in most US hospitals as a result of Joint Commission standards that require a mechanism for patients, family members, and employees to resolve ethical issues and provide ethics education. Ethics committees are best when they are interdisciplinary and contain representation from a wide range of stakeholders at the institution (e.g., physicians, nursing, social work, administration), and many include representatives from the community as well, such as a former patient, local clergy, or a philosophy professor from a nearby college. Additionally, most ethics committees have a lawyer as a member to assist in navigating the legal framework of cases and policies. Although ethical and legal issues are not the same, they are often intertwined, and ethics committees need to know, for example, the legal requirements for a surrogate decision-maker in order to effectively advise on the creation or revision of a surrogate decision-maker policy. Many ethics committees use an attorney from the community rather than the institution's legal counsel to avoid conflicts between the best ethical resolution of a particular case and the legal counsel's duty to minimize legal risk to the institution.

Ethics committee members are also diverse in terms of ethics training. If one does not have training in clinical ethics, it does not follow that one is not qualified to begin serving on an ethics committee. In fact, the majority of those who conduct ethics consultation do not have any formal ethics training [3]. It is essential to note that although most people who serve on ethics committees do not have formal clinical ethics training, it does not mean one should become complacent about one's own ethics training. In the resources section below, we recommend numerous educational opportunities, from one-day conferences to Master's degrees in bioethics.

Functions of an Ethics Committee

Education

The ethics committee is charged with the education of the members throughout the institution and, at times, patients and family members, and education is perhaps its most important function. In fact, if an ethics committee excels at education, it may prevent many ethics problems that would entail consultation requests from ever arising. For instance, if an ethics committee is effective at educating staff regarding the implementation of a power of attorney for healthcare, it may receive fewer requests regarding how to implement a power of attorney for healthcare. Also, if that same ethics committee explains that the person named as agent in the power of attorney for healthcare document is to make decisions as the patient would want them made, guided by the patient's values rather than by the agent's values, then requests for consults about this issue may decrease. Ethics committees also engage in education for the community that the institution serves. Educational outreach might include hosting ethics conferences to which the community is invited or simply providing education about why and how to complete a power of attorney for healthcare.

For the ethics committee to be effective in ethics education, however, it must prioritize education and not treat it as an afterthought. Some institutions have specific funds set aside to bring in an outside ethics expert, and most at least have an annual spot on the grand rounds schedule for a presentation sponsored by the ethics committee. Ethics committees should make the most of such opportunities to provide education to clinicians, patients, and families and also use the recommendations contained in consults as an opportunity to educate.

Another excellent continuing education opportunity for an ethics committee is to "assign" a pertinent article or reference for a discussion to be led by a member of the committee. Not only does this activity facilitate education, but it also invests the member who is presenting in the committee. Keeping records of the subject matter of ethics consultation requests can inform the educational endeavors of the committee. If a committee finds that the majority of requests for consultation focus on decisional capacity, for example, some education in that area would be of great value to the institution. Similarly, if the committee receives a large number of consult requests concerning advance directives, it might consider providing staff education on the institutional policy regarding advance directives.

Finally, an ethics committee should engage in regular self-examination as well, to identify any gaps in membership or needs for further education.

Policy Review

Most ethics committees develop, review, and provide advice for institutional policies that have an ethical impact. Common policies that an ethics committee might review include those addressing

DNR (do-not-resuscitate) status, surrogate decision-making, and advance directives. When institutions have a separate "institutional" or "organizational" ethics committee that addresses institutional policy issues, the ethics committee at such institutions should still review policies pertaining to such topics as ethics consultation.

Ethics committees need to be careful that they do not exceed their scope in reviewing policy. For example, a neurologist who serves on the ethics committee might disagree with the recommended tests in a brain death policy under review by the ethics committee. While that feedback might be important for the drafters of the policy, it is not the role of the ethics committee to weigh in on which tests should be used for determining brain death.

Consultation

Excellent available resources describe the process of ethics consultation [4], and each ethics committee will have its own approach to conducting ethics consultation. Nonetheless, there are some basic, important points concerning ethics consultation that are worth discussing in this chapter.

Ethics committees typically perform consultation according to four models: the team model, the ethics consultation service model, the full committee model, and the individual consultant model [5] (Table 18.1).

In the team model, a team of ethics committee members conducts the consultation and reports back to the committee, usually at the regularly scheduled meeting to keep the committee appraised of the nature of the consult and the recommendations made. In contrast, in the ethics consultation service model, the consult team includes people who are not members of the ethics committee. In both of these models, the entire committee does not weigh in on the recommendations prior to their issuance. For the full committee model, all the committee members (or, at least, those who can attend) participate in the consultation process. In the last model, an individual consultant, usually a member of the committee, performs the consultation. In all of these models, those present at the consult might be selected on an ad hoc basis or from the on-call schedule. We have served in all

Table 18.1 Ethics consultation models

Model	Involvement	Strengths	Weaknesses
Team	Some committee members	Different perspectives, more flexible than full committee, involves more committee members	Not as flexible as individual model, not as many perspectives as full model
Service	Some committee and non-committee members	Includes perspectives outside of the committee	External members may become disconnected from the ethics committee
Full	All available committee members	Broadest possible input	Difficult and slow to convene, large group may intimidate families or patients in a consult setting
Individual	One committee member	Fast and flexible	Lacks diverse viewpoints

four models and find that each has unique advantages and disadvantages. The decision regarding which model to employ should be guided by the qualification of the committee members and needs of the institution.

Regardless of the model employed, when a committee receives a request for an ethics consultation, the first question should be "What is the ethical question in the consult request?" This is important not only because it helps clarify and frame the matter of the consult (e.g., are we dealing with a question of decision-making capacity, a surrogate who is not making decisions appropriately, or both?) but because it can identify consult requests that may not be best addressed by the ethics committee. A common example might be a request for an ethics consultation in an end-of-life case that is better handled by the palliative care team, because the reason for the consult is not an ethical dilemma but, rather, a question surrounding the goals of care. Typically, ethics committee consultation focuses on ethical dilemmas, cases in which there is genuine uncertainty surrounding the ethically appropriate course of action. Ethics committees may also be requested to help in clarification or communication concerning an ethical concern. Ethics committees do not typically provide consultation for ethical violations, that is, cases in which someone is clearly behaving unethically and the person requesting the consult wishes action to be taken to correct the situation. Such a violation is better addressed elsewhere with the appropriate purview and function, such as the medical executive committee. It is important to be familiar with the spectrum of resources available at your institution because people who request an ethics consultation have genuine concerns and it is far better for everyone if the committee can refer people to the appropriate venue instead of simply stating that a particular case is not a case for the ethics committee.

An ethics committee might at times receive consult requests that, although technically not involving ethical dilemmas, may still be appropriate for some level of consultation. An example is the "moral distress" consult. A nurse might feel extreme frustration and moral distress over the way a case is managed. Although the ethics committee will not change the way the case is managed, its members might discuss the ethically relevant aspects of the case and listen to the nurse's concerns. Feeling heard may satisfy the nurse, and the case provides an opportunity for education.

Resources for Ethics Committee Members

An excellent starting place for resources for ethics committees is the American Society for Bioethics and Humanities (ASBH) and its publication, Core Competencies for Healthcare Ethics Consultation, Second Edition. ASBH also has numerous other resources for clinical ethics and ethics committees, as well as an annual conference and other smaller conferences that it sponsors and cosponsors. Additionally, an institution's or region's bioethics center can be an excellent resource for the ethics committee. Faculty from the bioethics center may already serve on the clinical ethics committee. Even if an institution does not have a bioethics center, it may have resources or training materials for ethics committee members. Additionally, ethics committee members may consider joining an ethics committee network, either as individuals or as an institution. Ethics committee networks, such as the Midwest Ethics Committee Network, the Maryland Healthcare Ethics Committee Network, and the Florida Bioethics Network, offer practical advice, sample policies, and the opportunity to network and learn from other regional ethics committees.

"Casebooks" can be an invaluable educational tool for a committee or individual as well [6, 7]. These books analyze some of the foundational cases in clinical ethics and provide a new ethics committee member with an understanding of those important cases and tools for deliberating about cases. The ethics committee can discuss such cases as a group for education sessions as well.

Consider also furthering your education in clinical ethics through attending a local seminar or a multiday ethics retreat or by earning a certificate or Master's degree in bioethics.

Key Concepts
- Ethics committees are multidisciplinary, containing representatives from a number of different fields.
- Ethics committees serve three functions: education, policy development and review, and consultation.
- Education is perhaps the most important of the ethics committee and should never be an afterthought.
- Ethics committees follow different models for consultation, and which model is followed depends on the needs of the institution.
- Ethics consultation recommendations in most institutions are just that, recommendations to the medical caregivers, patients, and families. The medical team makes the clinical decisions with input from the patient and family.
- Service on an ethics committee is enjoyable, thought provoking, meaningful, and often fun!

Words to the Wise
- You may receive "curbside consults" as a member of the ethics committee, that is, requests for advice on a case that are made in the hallway while you are consulting on another case, for example. Be mindful of whether the

(continued)

(continued)

issue is one that can be answered then and there (e.g., how do I activate a power of attorney for healthcare?) or by a formal ethics consultation.

- When receiving a request for an ethics consultation, prudent first questions to ask are "What is the central ethical question?" "What is the exact reason for the consult?" and "Is this consult request within the scope of the ethics committee?" If it is not, be sure to refer the person to the appropriate venue or committee.
- Sometimes an ethics consult request stems from moral distress, and despite the best efforts of the committee, the situation still ends poorly. At times the best you can offer is encouragement and a helpful ear.
- Commit to continuing ethics education: your own, the committee's, and the institution's.

Ask Your Mentor or Colleagues
- What kind of support is there, monetary and staffing, for the ethics committee?
- What model of ethics consultation does the committee follow? What was the rationale behind that choice?
- How much time does an ethics consult take, and how often will I be involved in consults?
- Which institutional policy, if any, sets out the purpose, scope, and composition of the ethics committee? To whom does the committee report? Where in the organization structure of the institution does the ethics committee reside?
- Will I have protected time to participate in the ethics committee and its work, and if so, what percentage of my time will be protected? If I do not have protected time, will my efforts be counted toward service to the institution in the promotion and tenure process?

References

1. Junkerman C, Derse A, Schiedermayer D. Practical ethics for students, interns, and residents: a short reference manual. 3rd ed. Hagerstown, MD: University Publishing Group, Inc.; 2008.
2. Lo B. Resolving ethical dilemmas: a guide for clinicians. 4th ed. Philadelphia, PA: Wolters Kluwer; 2009.
3. Fox E, Myers S, Pearlman RA. Ethics consultation in United States hospitals: a national survey. Am J Bioeth. 2007;7(2):13–25.
4. Aulisio M, Arnold R, Younger S, editors. Ethics consultation: from theory to practice. Baltimore, MD: The Johns Hopkins University Press; 2003.
5. Fletcher JC, Hoffmann DE. Ethics committees: time to experiment with standards. Ann Intern Med. 1994;120(4):335–8.
6. Pence G. Medical ethics: accounts of ground-breaking cases. 6th ed. Washington, DC: McGraw Hill; 2010.
7. Kuczewski M, Pinkus RL. An ethics casebook for: practical approaches to everyday cases. Washington, DC: Georgetown University Press; 1999.

How to Participate in Institutional Review Board Activities

19

Ann Freeman Cook and Helena Hoas

Institutional Review Boards (IRBs) serve as research oversight bodies charged with ensuring that risks to human subjects are minimized and reasonable, subject selection is equitable, and the informed consent documents are adequate. The regulations that underlie the protection of human subjects stem from the work of the Belmont Report, issued in 1978. This report was a response to the moral unease arising from revelations of the Tuskegee study and other problems such as a 1973 National Institutes of Health (NIH) recommendation that outlined the use of newly delivered live fetuses for medical research. In 1981, the IRB's responsibilities were codified in the Code of Regulations for Protection of Human Subjects, 45CFR 46, a regulation that covers the ethical conduct of biomedical, behavioral, and social research.

These regulations, referred to as the Common Rule, were further codified in 1991. Currently 19 federal agencies have adopted the Common Rule. Regulations from the Federal Drug Administration (FDA) and the Healthcare Insurance Portability Accountability Act (HIPAA) of 1996 added another layer of protection-related responsibilities. Since regulations continually

A.F. Cook, M.P.A., B.A., Ph.D. (✉)
Department of Psychology, The University of Montana,
341 Corbin Hall, Missoula, MT 59812, USA
e-mail: ann.cook@umontana.edu

© Springer International Publishing Switzerland 2016   269
L.W. Roberts (ed.), *The Associate Professor Guidebook*,
DOI 10.1007/978-3-319-28001-1_19

evolve, the Office of Human Research Protections (OHRP), a division within the Department of Health and Human Services (DHHS), offers guidance as a way to indicate the agency's current thinking on issues surrounding the protection of human subjects. Such guidance is viewed as a recommendation unless specific regulatory requirements are cited.

The Responsibilities of the IRB

The IRB provides review of new research and continuing review of existing studies at intervals appropriate to the degree of risk but not less than once per year. Fulfilling such oversight responsibilities requires that IRBs take into consideration the layers of regulation—including international, federal, sponsor, state, and institution—that govern the protection of human subjects. The work of the IRB is based on three core ethical principles. Respect for persons involves recognition of the personal dignity and autonomy of individuals and special protections for those with diminished autonomy. Beneficence entails an obligation to protect persons from harm by maximizing anticipated benefits and minimizing possible risks. Justice requires that the benefits and burdens of research be distributed fairly.

To fulfill these obligations, the IRB directs considerable efforts toward ensuring the informed and voluntary consent of those who are enrolled in research studies. According to regulations in the *US Department of Health and Human Services IRB Guidebook*, such consent must meet the "reasonable volunteer" standard which requires that "the extent and nature of information should be such that persons, knowing that the procedure is neither necessary for their care nor perhaps fully understood, can decide whether they wish to participate in the furthering of knowledge."

In order to fulfill regulatory requirements, IRBs are required to evaluate a study's research design, risks and benefits, subject selection, informed consent process, assurances of privacy and confidentiality, monitoring and observation, incentives for participation, and other regulations that may apply. An evaluation of each of these topics can entail considerable effort and, at times, controversy. A review of the informed consent process provides a good case in point. Although IRBs are expected to review the entire informed consent process, considerable attention can be focused on the informed consent document. Ideally, the document will be written in a way that truly enlightens the volunteer and so optimizes the likelihood of an informed decision.

It can be difficult, however, to impart information about research especially when enrolling persons who may have diminished cognitive capacities such as persons with Alzheimer disease or mental illness. Studies suggest that it is easy to enumerate the key elements of informed consent—full disclosure on the part of the researcher, adequate comprehension, and voluntary choice on the part of the subject—but difficult to accomplish. While people with recognized vulnerabilities may be disadvantaged when trying to make informed decisions, the authors' studies have shown that even well-educated participants may have little understanding of the research environment and tend to overestimate personal benefit and minimize potential risk. Thus IRB's members need to be vigilant in their efforts to discern the kinds of issues that can compromise participants' abilities to make informed and voluntary choices and then ensure that the study's research protocols address them.

Different Types of IRBs

When the IRB model was first developed, biomedical research was primarily conducted in academic medical centers. Indeed, as recently as 1994, the vast majority of biomedical research, including clinical research, was conducted in such settings. Each center or institution typically supported its own IRB(s), and the federal oversight guidelines and resources were developed with that institutional model in mind. Over time, new models such as independent or central IRBs, hospital IRBs, and community and tribal IRBs have become key players in the oversight system. Institutions have various protocols for approving studies that are conducted in their facilities or by their faculty. Depending on the kind of study and where it will be conducted, institutions may require approval by their own IRB, an independent or central IRB, or multiple IRBs.

An academician may be invited to serve on any one of these different types of IRBs. Some IRBs, when faced with challenging research protocols, use the services of consultants. Thus an academician may also be invited to serve as a consultant. When serving as either a member or consultant, it is important to clarify how one's knowledge and expertise will be reflected in the decisions made by the IRB.

What to Expect

The work that is required by the IRB can be time-consuming and at times frustrating. IRB members have reported that many hours, usually unreimbursed, are expended in reading research submissions and attending meetings. Meetings can be challenging as IRBs are required to be interdisciplinary and so draw on many different perspectives. Disagreements can easily arise. Applying ethical principles is not easy, especially because there is no single, overarching, super principle. It helps to expect that questions will be asked and ideas challenged and that differences of opinion may be voiced. When questions arise, it is not unusual to require resubmissions. Such resubmissions can be perceived as essential by the IRB members who are trying to optimize protection of human subjects but as frustrating delays by researchers who are trying to get studies under way.

Tension can arise because the very nature of the work creates challenges for both those who serve and those who submit protocols. It is important to be ethically attuned to the kinds of problems that can develop. While IRBs are charged with protecting human subjects, members report that they are also expected to protect the interests of researchers and their institutions and to advance science that benefits humanity. Ideally these goals are convergent, but in the real world, they can easily compete. Research can provide an important income stream for researchers and institutions. It can bring related benefits like fame and tenure and publications. The desire to receive such benefits can undermine efforts to fully protect human subjects.

Likewise, it can be difficult for IRBs to determine the extent to which a study truly benefits science and humanity. Many studies, especially those supported by the pharmaceutical industries, have commercial purposes that might be designed to primarily benefit the company rather than society. In a study conducted by the authors, IRB members lamented the lack of protocols or regulations that help them respond, in an ethical manner, when trying to address or resolve competing goals. The lack of guidance seemed to inhibit the ability of IRB members to tackle difficult ethical issues.

Overcoming Tensions

Recognizing and responding to issues that could compromise the protection of human subjects require training, introspection, and practical experience. Traditionally, there has been no uniform agreement about the kind of training in ethics that is needed in order to prepare persons for service on IRBs or for those who seek research careers. Thus ethical attunement often consists of "on-the-job" training. In an effort to institute a more uniform training, the Collaborative IRB Training Initiative (CITI) Human Subjects Training Program was developed in March 2000 through collaboration between the University of Miami and the Fred Hutchinson Cancer Research Center. This web-based ethics training underwent considerable expansion when the US Department of Health and Human Services announced its mandate for human subjects protection education. Currently IRB members, investigators, coinvestigators, and coordinators are required to complete the CITI training.

While such training provides a useful baseline, true ethical attunement requires the kind of introspection and reflection that comes from experience and further education. Most IRBs provide ongoing training programs for members and sometimes even for researchers in order to keep abreast of regulatory changes and emerging issues. Still, it can be hard to uphold the spirit of the regulations that underlies the protection of human subjects since regulations change, new challenges emerge, and the protectors (IRB members) and the protected (human subjects) may know little about one another.

Expanding One's Knowledge

The federal regulations identify special classes of people as vulnerable and requiring extra protection when enrolling in research studies. Such populations include, but are not limited to, prisoners, pregnant women, children and minors, persons with diminished capacities, terminally ill patients, and minorities. In addition, persons who may not initially seem to meet federal guidelines for vulnerability may bring vulnerabilities due to their life circumstances, beliefs, or values. Indeed, the authors' study showed that even well-educated participants based their decisions about participation on a pervasive level of trust—trust of the one who suggests participation (trusted physician), trust in the system (safe and not allowed if dangerous), trust in the product (new gold standard for treatment), and trust in the outcome (personal and humanitarian good). Thus they tended to gloss over or disregard any information in the consent documents that was inconsistent with such trust.

Such trust places a heavy moral burden on the shoulders of IRB members as they strive to protect human subjects but also strive to protect the interests of their own institutions or in the case of independent or central IRBs, the customers. Such burdens became apparent when IRB members who participated in the authors' study described how they approached two increasingly difficult issues: evaluation of the purpose of a study and disclosure and evaluation of researcher/institutional compensation. Members noted, for example, that the full purpose of the study was not always disclosed either to the IRB or to research participants. This occurs because some of the studies under review, mainly industry-funded studies, are designed to answer both scientific and commercial questions. The IRB review generally focuses on the scientific questions: Members noted that they are expected to assess the scientific merit of the study including the design, research protocols, and related issues such as safety, risk, and effectiveness but have less guidance about their role in assessing the nonscientific or commercial purposes of research. Members reported that it was not clear whether the IRB should require transparency about commercial purposes, if or how such purposes should influence the assessment of a study's scientific merits, whether research participants should be informed of commercial purposes, or how commercial purposes should be evaluated when considering the study's potential benefits to society.

Given the lack of guidance, most IRB members reported that information about the commercial purpose of a study was not "on the table" during the review process. Some IRB members reported a nagging sense that certain kinds of studies were not necessarily meritorious or truly beneficial to society; some members also suspected that participants may well want to be informed of commercial purposes before agreeing to enroll in a study. Indeed some members even reported that they themselves would certainly want to be informed of commercial purposes before participating in a study. Most noted, however, that any consideration of commercial purposes would remain "off the table" until regulatory guidance stipulates otherwise. Most IRB members also reported a lack of guidance about disclosure and discussion of researcher and institutional compensation; they noted that it was unclear what should be disclosed, to whom, or how. While all the IRBs vigorously examine and debate the compensation provided to research participants, most of the IRBs represented in this study did not request or receive detailed information about the study budget and so knew little about the amounts of researcher and institutional compensation.

Special Contributions of Persons with Medical Training

Persons with medical training bring unique perspectives and experiences to the IRB's deliberations about how to both optimize protection and achieve enlightened volunteers. Such training is especially helpful when assessing the purpose of the study, the potential for risk and the potential magnitude of harm posed by participation in a research study. Types of harm that are addressed via the informed consent form include physical, psychological, social, legal, and economic.

All of these areas for potential harm can be difficult for IRB members to assess. Examples of psychological, social, or behavioral harm can include emotional distress, psychological trauma, invasion of privacy, embarrassment, loss of social status, and loss of employment. Evaluating the magnitude of harm requires consideration of the duration, severity, and irreversibility of the research procedures. The IRB is tasked with performing a complicated risk-benefit analysis whereby risks to participants and the magnitude and probability of harm are balanced with the anticipated benefits to participants and the importance of the knowledge to be gained.

Making a Difference

The expectations and challenges discussed in this chapter offer insights as to why the work of the IRB is so important and why persons who serve in academic medicine can contribute significantly to that work. Such persons can encourage forthright discussions of the scientific value of the research as well as the needs, values, expectations, and vulnerabilities that participants may bring to the research enterprise. Such discussions in turn support the sustenance of an ethically attuned research environment, one that meets both the letter and the spirit of the regulatory guidance for protecting human subjects.

Words to the Wise
- Plan to attend scheduled meetings and be sure to arrive at the meeting on time.
- Be prepared to participate in "on-the-job" training activities.
- Ask questions that give insight into participant expectations and values and how they may influence decisions to enroll: What does this look like if I am standing in the shoes of the participant? How would I advise my mother, my friend? Would I seek this for myself?
- Look for articles on topics like therapeutic misconception, participant assessment of risk, and strategies for obtaining informed consent to enhance understanding of the ethical problems that can accompany research.
- Membership requires an ongoing commitment to self-reflection: Know what you know and what you do not know.

Ask Your Mentor or Colleagues
- What were your most memorable successes or regrets when serving on an IRB?
- How will the department view my service on the IRB?
- What personal and professional considerations should be "on the table" when deliberating membership on the IRB?
- What additional training might help me make ethically informed decisions?
- What considerations should go into my decisions about joining different types of IBBs or serving as a consultant for an IRB?

How to Think About Money in Academic Settings

20

Marcia J. Cohen

Achievement and fulfillment in academic medicine is enhanced with a basic understanding of how the "business" of academic medicine works.

The Different Colors of Money

Every organization requires money to pay its expenses. In medical schools, the revenues come from a variety of sources, and each of these sources typically has an important set of designations or restrictions which must be followed in how the funds can be expended. Finance managers and administrators are careful to spend funds in accordance with each fund's designations and restrictions to avoid time-consuming rework, costly overruns, or loss of future funding. Understanding in advance the "color of the money" will help faculty avoid these pitfalls.

Funds may be *designated* to the exclusive use of an individual department, division, program, or individual faculty member. Funds may also be *restricted* to be used only for specific purposes, such as funds restricted by a donor to be used to support cancer

M.J. Cohen, M.B.A. (✉)
Stanford University School of Medicine,
291 Campus Drive, MC 5216, Stanford, CA, USA
e-mail: mjcohen@stanford.edu

© Springer International Publishing Switzerland 2016
L.W. Roberts (ed.), *The Associate Professor Guidebook*,
DOI 10.1007/978-3-319-28001-1_20

research or research grant funds to be used only for the project purposes described in the grant proposal. The following paragraphs describe the major types of revenues in medical schools and their distinctive designations and restrictions.

Clinical Revenues

Typically, the largest source of funds in a medical school is the clinical practice of the faculty physicians who provide patient care in affiliated hospitals and clinics. In FY2010, 52 % of the revenues at the 126 accredited schools of medicine came from patient fees and medical center support [1]. Even at the largest *research-intensive* medical schools, the faculty clinical practice generates 40–60 % of total revenues [footnote AAMC/LCME data]. In some academic medical centers, the faculty practice revenues are controlled through a separate nonprofit faculty practice organization, which issues paychecks directly to faculty for the work performed through the faculty practice. In other academic medical centers, the academic departments receive the clinical revenues for their faculty's activities related to patient care and medical direction. These clinical revenues are controlled by departments and divisions and are used to support the compensation of clinically active faculty and a portion of department and division administration. These revenues are usually designated to the departments whose faculty earned them.

Clinical revenues are the least restricted of medical school revenues and can be used to cross-subsidize nonclinical activities, including education, research, infrastructure, and administration. Thus, clinical revenues are the source of the infamous *Dean's Tax*, a tithing from clinical revenues to support the infrastructure and investment of the school's dean's office. The Dean's Tax rates, set by the medical school dean, range from 3 to 10 %. The Dean's Taxes typically are used to shift revenues from larger or more profitable clinical departments to activities such as education or research, which are not entirely self-supporting. Departments and divisions also retain a portion of clinical revenues to support the administrative activities associated with clinical operations and with residency and fellowship programs.

Research Revenues

The second largest source of revenues in a medical school is sponsored research revenues from research grant awards and contracts. These revenues are designated to a specific individual faculty member, called the *principal investigator*, and are highly restricted—they must be used to support the research plan described in the proposal and in accordance with the approved project budget and the terms of the grant or contract. They must also be spent in compliance with university policies governing sponsored research and with government agency policies, if the source of the funding is governmental.

There are two major categories of revenues in most research grants and contracts. The *direct revenues* constitute the larger component of the grant and contract and are used to cover the expenses associated with the research program described in the proposal. These direct expenses include a portion of the salary and benefits commensurate with the percentage of time spent on the project by the investigator(s), postdoctoral fellow(s), and other research staff, plus any materials, supplies, and equipment associated with the research project.

The second category of research revenues is the *indirect revenues*. The indirect revenues are calculated as a percentage of the direct revenues, at a rate, called the *indirect cost recovery rate*, negotiated between the sponsor and the institution of the investigator. Indirect cost recovery rate negotiations between institutions and government agencies are conducted every 2–3 years and are based on the actual costs incurred by the institution for the infrastructure and administrative overhead of research activities. Typical expenses included in the indirect cost calculation are, among other expenses, utilities, space maintenance, accounting and research administration units, information technology, libraries, and interest and debt service for research buildings and equipment. Typical indirect cost recovery rates at large research-intensive medical schools range from 40 to 69 % for sponsored research. The average rate for accredited medical schools was 52.14 % in 2010 [2]. Rates for instructional grants, including training grants, are usually 10 %. Private foundations and other nonfederal research sponsors may allocate no funding for indirect costs or offer the institution a reduced rate of up to 10 %.

These indirect revenues are retained by the university, or allocated to the medical school, to support the infrastructure costs of research. Once received by the organization, the indirect research revenues can be repurposed and reallocated for other unrestricted purposes, such as support for research cores or investments in new programs.

Sponsored research grants and contracts are awarded to the institution of the principal investigator. The institution accepts the awards or enters into the research contract agreeing to administer the funds in accordance with the sponsor's terms and conditions. Medical schools or their parent universities are careful to administer the awards in accordance with these rules because a major infraction can bring sanctions across all the institution's research awards from that agency.

State Funds, Operating Budget allocations

Most medical schools receive an allocation of revenues for general operations either from state funds, if they are a public institution, or from the parent university, if a private institution. The state funds and university allocations are often reallocations of the tuition revenues received from medical students. These funds are primarily intended to pay for teaching and education program direction but are usually unrestricted and are also used to fund administrative support for teaching programs and faculty. A variety of formulae are used to allocate these funds to academic departments. Sometimes based on historical budget lines, many medical schools are revising their allocation formulae to track more closely the teaching effort of faculty. Even in major public institutions, the percentage of medical school revenues is small—in the range of 5–10 % or less.

Expendable Gift Revenue

Philanthropy comes in two distinct types—gifts, which are intended to be spent entirely, and endowments, which are invested by the institution and generate annual income for the donor's stated purposes (more on endowment income below).

Gift and endowment revenues are usually restricted and designated. The donor specifies the purpose(s) of the gift and often targets specific faculty recipients who will control the expenditure of the funds in accordance with the donor's intent. For example, a typical gift designation might be, "For the purpose of Dr. X's research program in acute lymphocytic leukemia." Gift funds often come through the institutional or the school development officers who work with the donor to craft a suitable donor agreement to ensure that the donor's wishes are adequately documented. Gifts typically fund only the direct costs of programs or services (see above discussion of direct costs under research revenues) but may also be general enough to cover the costs of administering the program or other closely associated infrastructure costs, such as equipment or space.

Foundations that seek to make large gifts typically request proposals outlining the plan and budget for how the gift will be expended. Most medical schools and parent universities have an administrative official who reviews all gifts to ensure that the funds coming into the institution are clearly categorized as "gift" or "grant." The lines distinguishing gifts and grants are blurry, but gifts do not typically require scientific or financial status reports, nor do they require the return of unexpended funds, as grants often do. Grants are charged indirect cost recovery and administered more closely to ensure that the budget is followed.

Donors do not typically require follow-up to ensure that funds have been spent in accordance with their wishes, nor do they specify a time horizon for the expenditure of their gift funds. But if they do follow up, institutions want to be able to demonstrate that the funds have been used well—to encourage more philanthropy from that donor and to avoid any appearance of impropriety, which may affect other giving.

Changes to the restrictions on gift funds are difficult, but not impossible. Institutional officials may contact donors to request a change in the restriction or designation. If the donor is deceased, then they may approach the donor's descendants. If no family is alive, the institution may petition the court to change the restrictions. There is a risk to each of these avenues for changing restriction—the donor, his or her family, or the court may decide that the institution can no longer carry out the donor's wishes, or the alternative proposed is not worthy, and instead of changing the designation, the court can withdraw the funds from the institution.

Endowment Income

Donors with the means to make large gifts may consider donating an endowment. Similar to expendable gifts, donors place restrictions and designations on these endowments. Because of the large size, endowments are usually set up to support an entire research or education program or a professorship. The size of a professorship is set by the institution (usually $2–$4 million) and is awarded to a faculty member to support his or her compensation and benefits and associated costs, such as administrative support and research expenses.

The initial money received for an endowment is called the endowment *principal*. Institutions pool individual endowment principal into larger pools for the purpose of managing these investments. The size of the endowment and its annual income is based on the number of shares "purchased" in the merged endowment pool and the average share price when the original endowment was established. The institution's governing body (e.g., the Board of Trustees) sets the annual income per share, which is typically in the range of 4–6 % of the current value of the endowment.

Once the endowment has been established, the value of the endowment principal can increase and decrease based on the results of the investment returns of the merged endowment pool. The original (or "permanent") endowment principal cannot be spent, but growth in the endowment that has accumulated over a number of years may be "invaded" if required to pay out the annual income set by the governing board. The current value of the endowment principal is reported at its current *market value*, and the annual income per share is typically set at a percentage of the market value at a specific point in time.

Institutions can also establish another type of endowment, called a *quasi endowment* or a *fund functioning as endowment* (FFE). Universities, medical schools, or departments may establish these quasi endowment funds to ensure an ongoing annual stream of funding for a specific purpose. These endowments follow all the same financial rules as regular endowments, but the endowment principal may be liquidated by the institution if financial needs change.

Other Miscellaneous Unrestricted Funds

Medical schools and departments have a myriad of other possible unrestricted revenues. These revenues include patent royalties from the licensing of faculty intellectual property, sales of special education programs and services, and revenues from auxiliary enterprises, such as fees generated from conferences, recreation facilities, rental properties, and contracts for special clinically related services at offsite locations.

Often these extra, unrestricted revenues are important sources of subsidy for education and research programs, pursued vigorously by department or school leadership, and carefully guarded to provide flexibility in covering the inevitable deficits and meeting financial commitments.

Fund Accounting

With so many different types of revenues, how do accountants track the restrictions and ensure appropriate expenditure of these funds?

Accounting systems in academic medical centers are based on principles of "fund accounting." Each unique revenue source (e.g., the clinical account for the surgical oncology faculty practice, the NIH grant for Dr. X, or the gift from Donor X for arthritis research) is set up as a separate fund which has restrictions recorded somewhere in the institution's financial records. Individual funds are given unique identifiers, including letters and numbers (e.g., ABDC-55057-123). Expenses are charged to individual funds using this unique identifier.

All expenses, including employee compensation, equipment, and supplies, must be charged to at least one fund. However, many expenses are split based on responsibility and charged to more than one fund because the expense benefited more than one program area. For example, the salary of a faculty member who spends 1 day in her surgical oncology clinical practice, 1 day teaching medical students, and 3 days on a sponsored research program may be expensed as follows:

- 20 % to the fund for surgical oncology's clinical practice
- 20 % to the fund for the surgery department's operating budget
- 60 % to the fund for the grant supporting the research program

At the end of each month, quarter, and fiscal year, financial reports detailing revenues and expenses for individual funds can be prepared to ensure that expenses do not exceed revenues. Monthly or quarterly review of financial reports is typical for all funds that are being actively spent. Many departments require projections of future revenues and expenses based on historical spending patterns through the end of the fiscal year or program period. Due to the restrictions on how individual funds can be spent, this active monitoring of revenues, expenses, and future projections is key to inform faculty and academic leadership of potential problems ahead, while there is still time to contain costs or search for alternate sources of funds.

Annual Budgeting

Medical schools, through their department and program units, prepare annual budgets of expected revenues and expenses in the coming fiscal year. This annual budget process is important for a number of reasons, including the concomitant budget negotiations that occur between dean's offices and departments, between hospital(s) and school, and between university and school. At the department level, one of the important objectives of the annual budget process is to estimate the costs of faculty compensation (usually the largest expense component) and the sources of funding in the coming year. Faculty may be queried about their outstanding sponsored research proposal pipeline, and the likelihood of new research awards, as well as the amount of time in patient care activities. At the department level, balancing the projected costs with projected sources of revenues to achieve at least a breakeven or better for the next budget year is the responsibility of the department chair along with the business manager. This is often done in conjunction with salary setting for the next year, since in most medical schools, awarding salary increases is dependent upon having available funds to support higher salaries.

Faculty members should find out when and how the local budget process is performed. Preparing any requests (such as those for new program initiatives) months in advance of the upcoming budget cycle will provide more opportunity to have the requests considered in the budget projections. Presenting requests in categories that fit the department or school budget format may also be helpful, for example, salary and benefits for each employee and itemizing non-salary expenses in the appropriate categories (telecommunications, materials and supplies, and meals and entertainment are typical categories in these budgets).

Commitments and Commitment Tracking

In addition to the annual budget process, most schools and departments track the commitment of funds that may span multiple budget years. Typical commitments include start-up funding for a new faculty's research program, a percentage of faculty salary over multiple years to provide specific services, or support for part of an equipment purchase if the investigator is successful in obtaining grant funding for the remaining costs.

If medical school or department leadership makes a financial commitment to you, you should ensure that the commitment is clearly stated in writing, and a copy is provided to the department business manager. At a minimum, it is good practice to estimate the total dollar amount of the commitment, estimates of annual allocations (which will facilitate budgeting), and what types of expenses will be covered by the commitment. The commitment may also be time limited, for example, the chair commits $50,000 per year for 3 years to support a new research program; any remaining funds not spent at the end of 5 years will return to the chair. This clarity incentivizes the expenditure of the funds and avoids unnecessary and unpleasant wrangling about remaining fund balances. At the end of each year, it is good business practice to provide faculty with the remaining balances in commitments. Most schools and departments wish to honor all commitments, including those promised by previous administrations. However, faculty can assist this process by seeking clarity in writing for all commitments and requesting annual reconciliations of remaining balances.

Clinical Funds Flow

Funds flow is the common term for the methodology governing how money for patient-related services provided in the hospital or clinics is passed to the faculty practice plan or the clinical department, if there is not a separate faculty practice plan, or from the faculty practice plan to the clinical department.

The most common *funds flow* method is that the entity that bills for the physician professional fees passes all revenues collected from these bills to the entity responsible for paying the faculty physician compensation. Often there are carve-outs before the revenues are passed for expenses, such as billing fees and other management services, the Dean's Tax, and the costs of clinic expenses related specifically to faculty practices.

Another *funds flow* method used in medical schools is based on physician payments per work RVUs, where the payment rate per work RVU is negotiated between the hospital and the school or department. Academic medical centers are also adding incentives and disincentives to these payment methods for patient satisfaction scores and quality measures.

Another component of funds flow is the support payments, typically from the hospital to departments, for medical direction or on-call coverage services provided by faculty physicians. Hospitals may also backstop the costs of new physician recruitment; typically, these last for up to 3 years, during which time the new physician builds a practice to a level that is self-sustaining.

Conclusion

Medical schools and departments are funded by a variety of revenue sources, each with unique designations and restrictions. Academic business managers and faculty leadership are careful to spend funds according to their restrictions in order to avoid costly rework and the potential of jeopardizing future funding from government, university, or donor sponsors. The annual budget process brings this all together in a skillful balancing exercise to plan how the next year's projected revenues will cover projected expenses. Important to individual faculty or programs are commitments made by leadership that span more than 1 year. Having clearly written commitments is an important step in securing funding and avoiding future disagreements or disappointment. Funds flow is the common term for the methodology governing how money generated from patient-related activities is passed to the school or department. Funds flow methods differ at various academic medical centers but are typically based on the professional fees collected or on a payment-per-work RVU method.

Words to the Wise
- Plan your potential funding needs several years in advance to ensure that you will have the funds available to pursue your academic goals.
- Discuss your plans and potential fund sources with your department business manager.
- Include an annual inflation factor in future years.
- Understand the restrictions of the funding sources you have. Plan carefully how to justify the expenditure of any restricted funds provided to you, matching the expenses with the restrictions of the fund.
- If you are using gift or endowment income funds, establish a relationship with the donors, and provide timely reports on your work and achievements. Your development officer(s) may help you with these relationships, and ultimately this may lead to more funding.
- Review your accounts on a regular basis; if not monthly, then at least quarterly.
- Work with your business manager or financial analyst to project future expenditures and plan ahead. Ideally, your efforts on a particular project or program will be completed when the funding runs out. Further, your ability to sustain programs with new sources of funding will be greatly enhanced through careful financial projections and anticipation of when more funding will be needed.

Ask Your Mentor or Colleagues
- I am interested in understanding the major sources of revenues for our School of Medicine and for our department. Can you share with me the School of Medicine's annual financial report?
- Can you share with me the department's annual financial report and annual budget?
- From where do the funds for my compensation and program funds come? How much of the physician fees generated from my practice are returned to the department (division)?
- (If you have a start-up package) May I review with you the sources of funding for my start-up package? I would like to understand if any of the funds are restricted.
- With whom should I work on receiving regular financial reports on my accounts? Are there any tips you have for understanding these reports?

References

1. Source: LCME Part I-A Annual Medical School Financial Questionnaire (AFQ), FY2010. Prepared by AAMC June 2011. Contact: Kajal Nayyar, Senior Research Analyst, Medical School and Faculty Studies. (202) 478–9913 or knayyar@aamc.org. © Association of American Medical Colleges 2011. All rights reserved.
2. Federal Negotiated Facilities and Administrative (F&A) Rate: Source: LCME Part I-A Overview of Organizational and Financial Characteristics Survey. © Association of American Medical Colleges 2011. All rights reserved.

Further Reading

Mallon William T, Vernon David J, and colleagues at the AAMC. The handbook of academic medicine—how medical schools and teaching hospitals work. 2nd ed. Washington, DC: Association of American Medical Colleges; 2008.

How to Negotiate

21

Mickey Trockel

A popular dictionary definition of negotiation is "to confer with another or others in order to come to terms or reach an agreement" [1]. The goal of negotiation is to reach an agreement, and the basic process of negotiation is back-and-forth communication. Within this basic definition of negotiation falls a myriad of strategies, methods, and underlying goals, pressures, and ethical assumptions driving a large range of negotiation styles. An unenlightened perspective of negotiation may classify negotiation styles as hard or aggressive vs. soft or passive, or somewhere in between. Aggressive negotiators place high premium on the goals they are trying to obtain and discount the relationship costs associated with doggedly digging in their heels to defend the position they presume paramount. They are inflexible and not given to compromise.

Imagine a department head embracing this negotiation style when approaching senior faculty to discuss the need to increase revenue in order to rectify the department's precarious financial circumstances. She may approach a negotiation with faculty as an opportunity to convince them of the necessity and urgency to implement her plan to increase the number of patients each faculty

M. Trockel, M.D., Ph.D. (✉)
Department of Psychiatry and Behavioral Sciences, Stanford University,
401 Quarry Road, Stanford, CA, USA
e-mail: trockel@stanford.edu

© Springer International Publishing Switzerland 2016
L.W. Roberts (ed.), *The Associate Professor Guidebook*,
DOI 10.1007/978-3-319-28001-1_21

member must see in a week. When other faculty members suggest the correct strategy is to increase research funding and to engage in more fund-raising, she may feel her position of authority is being challenged and articulately discount these options as too slow and then comment: "The best academic physicians welcome increased opportunity to help patients and are able to do good research at the same time. Others aren't yet as motivated, but we can help them come around." Her comment suggests that those who oppose her perspective are lazy. The more others suggest opposing views, the more articulately and passionately she discounts them and the integrity of their authors. If she continues with her approach to negotiation and is eventually able to implement her plan, at least some of her faculty members are likely to begrudge the change and will look for an opportunity to defeat her or to get a new department head if they have the opportunity to do so.

Now imagine a department head with the same circumstances who embraces the opposite negotiation style, passive acquiescence to win favor with faculty, discounting the integrity of a viable solution to his department's financial problems. Although nobody is wildly enthusiastic about his proposal, some faculty are open-minded, understand the financial constraints, and are willing to give his plan a try. These members of the faculty say nothing when he suggests his plan to require every faculty member to increase clinical revenue from direct patient care. Others are clearly upset and insist on finding another solution. Those who oppose an increase in clinical revenue targets propose an alternative strategy of increasing department acquisition of NIH research funding. The department head is acutely aware of the risky business plan of betting the department's current fiscal integrity on uncertain NIH research funding that will take at least 1 year to procure even if a well-executed increase in grant writing is perfectly successful. However, he feels his relationship with faculty who oppose his views is of primary importance and wants to win points with them by giving their plan a try. Unfortunately, his points with these faculty members are likely to be far spent if 1 year later he must propose more drastic measures such as a pay cut or increased work hours in order to balance a then drowning department checkbook. And the dean may try to get a new department head if she has the opportunity to do so.

Most negotiations in any context and virtually all negotiations in the context of academic medicine take place within longer term interpersonal relationships and organizational structures. The long-term interpersonal relationship context makes both aggressive (hard) and passive (soft) negation styles more problematic. Any negotiation style that pits goals of getting what one wants from others against collegial relationships and organizational integrity has no place in academic medicine.

Foundations of Principled Negotiation

The enlightened view of negotiation is not the halfway point between the dysfunctional aggressive or passive extremes. Rather, an enlightened view of negotiation simultaneously and completely embraces the principles that protect the interests driving the negotiator's participation in the negotiation (respect for self) and those that uphold the importance of treating people—including opposing negotiators—with dignity, empathy, and equanimity (respect for others). Effective negotiation is grounded in mutualism, communication, preparation, self-knowledge, and self-observation. Our description of principled negotiation in this chapter leans heavily on a classic book on this subject—"Getting to Yes: Negotiating Agreement Without Giving In" [2]. We focus our discussion on the application of principled negotiation strategies in the context of a career in academic medicine. Adherence to these principles will increase your chances of good negotiation outcomes and good interpersonal relationship outcomes.

Separate Relationship Issues from Negotiated Issues

The weightiest outcome in most negotiations is the effect of the negotiation interaction on the long-term relationship of the negotiating parties. The specific issue at hand being negotiated will usually pale in comparison. In a negotiation over who gets a vacant cubicle of office space, a senior professor may be able to use his "rank" as the winning determinant of space allocation, overriding a more junior colleague's actual need driven by her current space limitation requiring three research assistants to share one cubicle. However, the cost of playing the "rank card" with no principled negotiation may be that subsequent collaboration with the more junior colleague will be soured, or perhaps not even possible without some effort to repair the relationship damage. Six months later when the department head announces a plan for construction of a new facility that solves critical space limitations for everyone, the victory over a single-cubicle stewardship becomes even hollower, while the relationship loss remains. Even when negotiating seemingly critical issues such as a new academic appointment, the relationship between the negotiators will usually prove to be the most important long-term outcome of the process. Failure to recognize the importance of relationship factors can lead to bruised egos, inability to reach an agreement, resentment, and retaliation harmful to both parties. Nevertheless, placing a premium on relationship outcomes does not require dismissal of the substantive problem being negotiated.

It is essential to separate relationship issues from substantive problem issues. It is almost always possible to strive for positive relationship goals and substantive problem-solving goals, without losing sight of either in the negotiation process. If the professor discussed above had given due regard to his relationship with his more junior colleague, he may have taken time to explain the fact that he was anticipating a new center grant which would require extensive staffing while making an effort to understand his colleague's critical space needs.

When preparing for a negotiation, first decide on the relationship outcome you want to achieve; then decide on the specific issue outcome you want to achieve. During this planning stage, it is often useful to learn what you can about your negotiation partner's needs, ambitions, and circumstances. Then, practice arguing the issues you plan to negotiate from the vantage point you believe represents your negotiation partner's perspective. Keep in mind your negotiation partner's basic human needs for safety, social support and love, respect, autonomy, and mastery [3]. Then, reflect on your needs, ambitions, and circumstances. Thoroughly reflect on the question: "Why are the relationship and the specific negotiation outcomes important to you in this negotiation?" After you have reflected on your negotiation partner's interests and yours, you will be far more prepared to work towards protecting both.

Identify Interests Rather Than Fixate on Positions

Focus on interests underlying hoped for negotiation outcomes makes it easier to achieve an agreement while respecting the long-term relationship between negotiators. Conversely, focus on positions pits the needs of one party against the other arbitrarily and makes it difficult to separate the specific negotiation problem from the people involved in the negotiation.

To illustrate some of the pitfalls of focus on positions, consider the failed negotiation between a psychiatry department head and an applicant she was trying to recruit to fill an open associate professorship in her department. The department invested approximately $3000 to fund the interview and site visit, in addition to dozens of hours donated by faculty and support staff spent on the process. The department head carefully examined the financial position of the department, including the compensation amount current faculty in her department were receiving. She determined she could offer $189,000 to the applicant, with no flexibility to negotiate for a higher salary. The applicant, aware he may be receiving an offer, carefully considered his current salary at a more prestigious institution where he was an assistant clinical professor. He calculated his "bottom-line" salary by considering his current salary and his current call schedule compared to the call schedule he had learned he would assume at the university wanting to recruit him. His current salary was $155,000, to which he added $50,000, to represent the value he placed on being on call once per week at the smaller university department compared to once per month at his current larger institution. However, he wants to move to the new location—at least in part—because his fiancée has just accepted a very lucrative job in the area. Here is how the short telephone negotiation went:

Department head:	"We would like to offer you the associate professor position with our department. I can offer you $189,000 and the standard benefits package we have talked about."
Applicant:	"I liked what I saw when I came to visit, but I was expecting a more attractive financial offer."
Department head:	"How much were you hoping for?"
Applicant:	"Based on my current salary and circumstances, I'm hoping for $221,000."
Department head:	(Taken back by that figure as it exceeded her own salary by about $5000). "While we would like you to join our faculty, unfortunately, we really can only offer $189,000."
Applicant:	"My bottom line is $205,000."
Department Head:	"I really can't offer you more than $189,000."
Applicant:	(Surprised at the department head's inflexibility) "Can I sleep on it and call you in the morning?"
Department head:	"Sure. We'll look forward to your call."

The next day, the applicant feels he cannot accept the offer based on the principle that "to take a pay cut would be a career-backslide." He calls the department head and graciously declines the offer. Although simplistic, this brief dialogue illustrates some of the problems inherent in a negotiation focused on positions. The department head does not arrive at an understanding of the applicant's interests in obtaining compensation he deems equivalent to his current position with another university at a lower academic rank, adjusted for the difference he perceives in call frequency. Nor does she arrive at an understanding of the high monetary value the applicant has placed on having a lighter call schedule. The applicant does not seek to understand the department head's motivation in recruiting him nor her interest in fairness to other faculty and the financial integrity of the department. Neither is happy with the brief negotiation outcome, and both were left with somewhat more negative views of each other following the negotiation impasse.

The outcome may have been different if both the applicant and department head had focused on the interests rather than on inflexible positions. The department head may have asked questions such as the following: Although you would be on call more frequently here than where you currently work, how do you think call nights here compare with call nights where you are now? What do you feel you are giving up if you are on call once per week vs. once per month? How does pressure to publish papers where you are now compare with the goal of one paper every 2 years in our department? What besides salary and call schedule weigh in to your decision?

The applicant may have disclosed the way he arrived at his bottom-line salary calculation by considering his interests in compensation and in a light call frequency. He may have asked the department head questions such as the following: What keeps you from being able to offer more? What besides affordable compensation do you consider important to the department when you negotiate a new academic contract with an applicant? What about me in particular do you consider valuable enough to your department to offer me this job? After discussing the answers to these and other questions focused on both parties' interests driving their part in the negotiation, the applicant and department head will be well positioned to move forward. Specifically, armed with understanding of their own and each other's interests, they will be able to work together to creatively think of ways to meet those interests within the financial and other organizational constraints framing their effort to reach an agreement about compensation and other details of a new appointment contract. In addition, sincerely seeking to understand each other's interests will facilitate early relationship building that may benefit both directly as they work together following agreement on the terms of a new academic contract. Even if the applicant does not join the department head's faculty, the more thoughtful negotiation process is likely to lead to better feelings on both sides of the negotiation table that could pay reputation dividends later in the relatively small world of academic psychiatry.

Identify Several Options to Generate Mutual Benefit Before Deciding

A creative search for solutions that would serve both the department head's and the applicant's interests may make it possible for both to benefit significantly. Would the applicant (board certified in forensic psychiatry) consider doing some forensic psychiatry consultation for the department to justify a pre-negotiated stepped increase in salary contingent on his revenue productivity? Could a night-shift hospitalist be hired to reduce call schedule demands for all faculty members? What would the applicant consider to be a fair salary if he were relieved of all call responsibilities? Does the department have any way of offering housing purchase assistance that is not part of the base salary? Is there a mechanism to create bonus income from clinical revenues in excess of a minimum quota? If the applicant's job duties include securing funding for research, is there a mechanism for increasing salary based on successful research grant funding? On the applicant's end, there may be ways to obtain benefits that may be worth a somewhat lower salary, such as office space, support staff, greater clinical autonomy, and a greater ratio of teaching and research vs. clinical time allocation.

In order to generate a sufficient number of possible solutions to key negotiation problems, it is essential to uphold curiosity and free discovery while suspending judgment. When negotiating an offer for an academic appointment, it may be helpful to take a time-out to generate alternatives in another location or to meet with other faculty members separate from discussion with the applicant in order to reduce inhibition during the idea-generating step. Suspending the assumption of fixed resources is also important. There may be creative ways that addition of a new associate professor could increase department revenues in a way that benefits all. Focus on interests and creative ideas to meet interests of both parties as much as possible will facilitate decision making.

During the decision-making step, principled negotiators will insist on outcomes based on objective standards, rather than based on eloquent arguments or passionately held positions.

Insist on Outcomes Based on Objective Standards

In the above example, the applicant focused on his position of a bottom-line salary. Logically, he based his counter offer of $221,000 simply by doubling the distance between his bottom line and the department head's offer, hoping she would "at least" meet him half way. He didn't articulate the principles he felt underscored his hope for a higher salary (his current salary plus $50,000 to account for the difference in call schedule intensity). The department head did not disclose the reasoning behind the amount she offered, which was based on the salary range of her current faculty members and current national academic psychiatry salary ranges. Other objective criteria the department head might have considered during negotiation of salary could have included call frequency in other departments offering similar salary compensation and cost of living differences between the new location and the applicant's current location. Insisting on outcomes based on objective standards helps negotiators separate people from the issues they are negotiating, which can help protect long-term relationships in the process.

Attention to the relationship context of negotiation, focus on creative ways to serve the interests of both parties, and basing decisions on objective criteria rather than on positions will enhance the quality of the negotiation process and associated outcomes. Nevertheless, even the most principled negotiators will run into problems that threaten the negotiation process and outcomes.

Navigating Negotiation Barriers with Grace and Purpose

Troubleshooting the entire breadth of problems encountered during negotiation is beyond the scope of this chapter. Here, we focus on active listening and dealing with difficult emotions. We then briefly discuss considerations for negotiating when power between you and your negotiation partner is not equal. We conclude with advice on how to improve your negotiation skills over time, including a list of books for further learning on the topic.

Identifying and Managing Communication Problems

Misunderstanding is perhaps the most common communication problem. Just a slight change in intonation or volume can change meaning. Consider the simple change in placement of a pause, represented in writing by a comma: "She's an amazing clinician sometimes" vs. "She's an amazing clinician, sometimes." The message heard often differs from that intended by its author. The best strategy for preventing or ameliorating misunderstanding is active listening. Active listening also attenuates the natural tendency to focus on what to say next while your negotiation partner is speaking. Almost everyone has stumbled on this communication barrier on at least a few occasions and will have learned by personal experience that we have limited capacity to simultaneously listen to understand someone else while focusing intently on fabricating an articulate next response. Tenaciously avoid the temptation to plan your next line when your negotiation partner is speaking. Carefully listen. Then, verbally summarize with comments like "Let me see if I understand you. You need the office space because you currently have three research assistants in one cubicle." This gives your negotiation partner a chance to clarify. Then, after listening and seeking to understand, you have a better chance of being understood when you explain your vantage point. "I see how that is difficult. Unfortunately, if I do not get the space, I will not be able to hire additional staff for the new grant-funded project that starts next week because I already have three staff members making shift-rotation use—two at a time—of both the cubicle spaces I have allocated to my lab currently." Misunderstanding and perceived pressure to come up with a persuasive next response will become more prevalent when the emotional intensity of a negotiation increases. Managing emotions is a critical negotiation skill.

Managing Emotions in Negotiations, Yours and Theirs

Be not hasty in thy spirit to be angry: for anger resteth in the bosom of fools. Ecclesiastes 7:9.

As the above ancient proverb implies, anger seems to compromise intelligent action. Negotiators with high anger and low feelings of compassion towards each other achieve fewer gains during negotiation and are less likely to want to work together in the future [4]. Consider your own experience. If you are like most people, you have not experienced your best thoughts, words, or actions when you were angry. In contrast, you are likely to recognize that many of your words and actions when you were most angry are those you have regretted most. Like anger, anxiety can also jeopardize favorable negotiation outcomes [5]. Strong anger or strong anxiety can block communication or create turbulent communication, which causes misunderstanding, perceived or actual aggressive interactions, intimidation, defensiveness, or unproductive passivity. The associated negotiation outcomes can be unhappy for everyone involved.

Be aware of your emotions before and during negotiation. When you notice you are experiencing an unpleasant emotion, label the emotion. The simple act of labeling the emotion you are experiencing in the moment can initiate prefrontal cortex attenuation of amygdala-driven emotional intensity [6]. It may also be helpful to use "I feel" statements [7]. If you are feeling anxious during a negotiation, stating this openly may help reduce the intensity of your own anxiety and will welcome similar response from your negotiation partner. Imagine the relationship-soothing effects of such open communication modeled by a department head during negotiation with a long-time donor to the department's general research fund. "As we talk about the reduction in the amount of your annual donation and associated reduction in our research program, I am feeling a bit nervous. I am guessing this may not be an easy conversation for you either." Making emotions explicit allows people to deal with strong feelings openly, rather than tripping over them in a dysfunctional, emotionally laden communication process. Being aware of your emotions and perceptive of your negotiation partner's emotions can prevent negotiators from losing perspective and making serious mistakes [8]. Openly acknowledging your emotions when you feel passionately about something may also help you be understood and make your point, which can allow you to make strong emotions work for you rather than against you during negotiation. It is equally important to recognize and acknowledge your negotiation partner's emotions. Being accurately perceptive of a negotiation partner's emotions correlates with higher performance in achieving favorable negotiation outcomes [9].

If you notice your negotiation partner is becoming angry, use the disarming communication technique of openly acknowledging the element of truth in what you are being accused of [7]. For example, consider the example of an internal medicine applicant who has been negotiating an appointment contract during the past week. He is holding strongly to his interest in compensation equal to the average amount paid to other equally ranked academic internists. His potential new department head seems exasperated as, in a frustrated tone of voice, he fires off, "You cannot seem to see beyond the narrow scope of the base salary amount to consider the other very attractive aspects of our offer, including a tenure appointment and guaranteed 50 % time research funding for the next three years." The temptation when feeling attacked is to become defensive, which could lead the applicant to fire back, "I just want to be compensated fairly, commensurate with other equally ranked academic internists." If he keeps his cool and is able to use the disarming technique, he may instead respond with something like "I see your point. You are absolutely right; during the last 30 min of our conversation I have focused exclusively on salary amount and have not even acknowledged the generous aspects of your current offer, like the excellent guaranteed research funding and lab space you are offering me. While I would still like to agree on a base salary commensurate with other equivalently ranked academic internists, I am feeling embarrassed that I have failed to acknowledge the very generous aspects of your current offer as you have described them during the past 30 min of our conversation." In both cases, the applicant appropriately focuses on objective salary criteria. However, adding a disarming comment to address his potential new department head's frustration during the negotiation process may make it easier to reach an eventual agreement and is likely to help the applicant with her goal of establishing a good relationship with her potential new boss.

Communicating an empathetic understanding of your negotiation partner's concerns and use of sincere complements when appropriate are also important communication skills that facilitate relationship bridges during the negotiation process. Nevertheless, even with good communication skills, it may be more challenging to achieve an optimal negotiation process or outcome when the balance of power is markedly unequal between negotiators.

Tips for Negotiation When Your Position of Power Is Not Equal

Ideally, negotiation involves side-by-side partnership rather than head-on confrontation. A metaphor representation of this concept is a boat with a motor on a freely moving shaft in back and a steering wheel connected to a rudder in front. Both must be manned to move the negotiation boat forward. However, when one negotiation party seems to have control of both ends of the boat, motivation to work together to navigate a negotiation process may be less obvious. This can occur, for example, when a department head is considering "negotiating" an increase in faculty clinical workload to offset emerging budget difficulties.

A simple negotiation tool that can help under-empowered negotiators in such circumstances is knowing their best alternative to a negotiated agreement (BATNA) [2]. In the above example, if a productive assistant professor can obtain an offer for employment at a nearby prestigious university, her BATNA will be very empowering. For others, a BATNA of nonacademic employment may feel empowering when discussing clinical quotas with the department head during a faculty meeting. Some research evidence suggests having an identified BATNA may increase productive assertiveness during negotiation [10]. In the context of a negotiation with the department head about clinical productivity quotas, faculty who have identified their BATNA are likely to feel more empowered and will probably be more likely to suggest creative alternatives to increasing their clinical quotas, if they feel another alternative should be sought.

Motivation to engage in egalitarian negotiation from the perspective of the empowered negotiator may be in short supply when holding a significant power advantage. The temptation to efficiently compel rather than struggling to patiently persuade is an ever-present temptation faced by all people who hold any position of power over others. The developmental growth and relationship costs of giving in to this temptation can be catastrophic. Whether a parent or head of state, compelling compliance can suffocate autonomy, stifle creativity, and bruise relationships beyond repair. Leadership in academic medicine affords no exception to these basic principles. Although there are some circumstances when forced compliance is warranted (e.g., when a toddler is running towards oncoming traffic, a parent may need to forcibly change the toddlers trajectory.), whenever negotiation is appropriate, opting for unilateral compulsion may yield more rapid change in the short term, but the cost may be unacceptable in the long term. Carefully honing negation skills is a worthwhile endeavor for academic medical professionals of all ranks.

Developing and Enhancing Your Negotiation Skills Over Time

Frequent practice coupled with self-monitoring of performance criteria is key to mastery of most skills, including those pertaining to negotiation. After each opportunity to negotiate, consider evaluating your own performance in implementing the four basic strategies of principled negotiation introduced in this chapter and described in detail in the book "Getting to Yes: Negotiation Agreement Without Giving In" [2]. In addition, consider evaluating your use of good communication skills during negotiation, using effective communication criteria such as those outlined by David Burns [7].

Words to the Wise

Strategies of principled negotiation [2]:

- Separate relationship issues from negotiated issues.
- Identify interests rather than fixate on positions.
- Identify several options to generate mutual benefit before deciding. Insist on outcomes based on objective standards.

Five elements of effective communication [7]:

- Ask additional questions to understand what your negotiation partner is thinking and feeling.
- Thought empathy (summary restatement of what was said) and feeling empathy (accurately reflecting back an understanding of emotions felt).
- The disarming communication technique. Sincere complements. "I feel" statements (stating the emotion you experience, without assigning blame).
- "I feel" statements (stating the emotion you experience, without assigning blame).

Ask Your Mentor or Colleagues

- What factors should I consider when evaluating an academic offer?
- What things do you wish you had considered when you negotiated your contract?
- What are the things that you are happy you did consider when you negotiated your contract?

References

1. Farlex. The Free Dictionary by Farlex; http://www.thefreedictionary.com/negotiate. Accessed 19 Nov 2012.
2. Ury W., Fisher, R. Getting to yes: negotiation agreement without giving in. 2nd ed. New York: Penguin Books; 1992.

3. Tay L, Diener E. Needs and subjective well-being around the world. J Pers Soc Psychol. 2011;101(2):354–65.
4. Allred KG, Mallozzi JS, Matsui F, Raia CP. The influence of anger and compassion on negotiation performance. Organ Behav Hum Decis Process. 1997;70(3):175–87.
5. Brooks AW, Schweitzer ME. Can Nervous Nelly negotiate? How anxiety causes negotiators to make low first offers, exit early, and earn less profit. Organ Behav Hum Decis Process. 2011;115(1): 43–54.
6. Hariri AR, Bookheimer SY, Mazziotta JC. Modulating emotional responses: effects of a neocortical network on the limbic system. Neuroreport. 2000;11(1):43–8.
7. Burns D, Aurbach A. Therapeutic empathy in cognitive-behavioral therapy: does it really make a difference? In: Salcovskis P, editor. Frontiers of cognitive therapy. New York, NY: The Guilford; 1996. p. 135–64.
8. Adler RS, Rosen B, Silverstein EM. Emotions in negotiation: how to manage fear and anger. Negotiation J. 1998;14(2): 161–79.
9. Elfenbein H, Foo M, White J, Tan H, Aik V. Reading your counterpart: the benefit of emotion recognition accuracy for effectiveness in negotiation. J Nonverbal Behav. 2007;31(4):205–23.
10. Magee JC, Galinsky AD, Gruenfeld DH. Power, propensity to negotiate, and moving first in competitive interactions. Pers Soc Psychol Bull. 2007;33(2):200–12.

Further Reading

Ury W. Getting past no: negotiating in difficult situations. New York: Bantam Books; 1991.
Ury W, Fisher R. Getting to yes: negotiating agreement without giving in. 2nd ed. New York: Penguin Books; 1992.

How to Read a Basic Budget

22

David J. Peterson

Throughout the course of an academic career in medicine, faculty will inevitably be asked to review and even construct a budget. Such a review could be in the context of evaluating the financial health and performance of a departmental or an institutional program. If research is a component of the academic career and the faculty member is the principal investigator, co-investigator, or one of key personnel on a grant, the faculty member will most certainly need to build a budget and track its performance and may even need to review a budget as a member of a review committee at the local or national level. Developing an understanding of budgets, then, is an important skill set for the academic faculty member to acquire.

More than a page of numbers, budgets tell a story. Regardless of the context for this story—be it clinical, educational, or research—knowledge of a few basic budgeting principles will contribute to the faculty member's confidence and success in both telling and understanding the story. Budgets can tell the reader how a program will be supported (revenue) and how the funds will be spent (expenses). Within these broad categories, budgets provide detail about how the funds will be earned and spent and on what they will

D.J. Peterson, M.B.A., F.A.C.M.P.E. (✉)
Department of Psychiatry and Behavioral Medicine, Medical College of Wisconsin, 8701 Watertown Plank Road, Milwaukee, WI, USA
e-mail: Peterson@mcw.edu

© Springer International Publishing Switzerland 2016   307
L.W. Roberts (ed.), *The Associate Professor Guidebook*,
DOI 10.1007/978-3-319-28001-1_22

be spent. Once a budget is established and a program is initiated, budgets can help measure performance by comparing actual revenue and expenses to those that were expected (budgeted).

Budget Basics

Although the format, platform, or audience for a budget can vary, the reviewer can rely on a basic set of traditions, conventions, and principles when evaluating a budget. These "generally accepted" principles are found in a national set of standards identified as Generally Accepted Accounting Principles, or GAAP. GAAP rules ensure a level of standardization and include such principles as "sincerity, consistency, continuity, and good faith" [1].

In its most simple form, a budget identifies the resources a program will require to fund the expenses necessary to support the program's goal. Resources—revenue—can come from a variety of sources. For example, revenue can be a direct award of departmental, institutional, or agency funds; revenue can be drawn from philanthropy, public, or private sector grants; or revenue can be generated from professional fees derived from the clinical services or medical direction provided, to name a few.

Expenses are usually grouped into categories such as personnel costs (salaries), fringe benefits, general supplies and expense, equipment, and travel. Rent for the space the program occupies is often included in a budget except in the instance of federally funded and other extramural research where a factor for "facility and administrative" costs (also known as "indirect costs") is calculated on the total proposed direct costs in the budget. [Direct and indirect costs are described in more detail later in this chapter in the section labeled "A Federal Twist on Research and Other Program Budgets"]. Figure 22.1 is an illustration of a simple revenue and expense budget. Budgets are often accompanied by a narrative description, describing the overall intent of the project or program, and justifying, if necessary, the revenues and expenses proposed.

All budgets identify the revenues and expenses of a project, program, or organization over a period of time. Time is generally measured as a 12-month period referred to as a *"fiscal year."*

Academic Medicine Department/Program
School of Medicine
University of State
July 1, 20XX - June 30, 20X+1

	Budget
Revenues	$ 135,000
Expenses	
Faculty Salaries	75,000
Staff Salaries	10,000
Fringe Benefits	25,500
Supplies & Expense	10,000
Other	5,000
Subtotal Expenses	$ 125,500
Total Profit (Loss)	$ 9,500

Note: Generally accepted practices in budget presentations include a descriptive header, the period that the budget covers, dollar signs at the beginning and after each line for a subtotal or total, and a double underline indicating a final total.

Fig. 22.1 Sample revenue and expense budget

Fiscal years can start at any time during a calendar year, but as a general rule, once the fiscal year is defined, the start and end dates of the fiscal year need to be consistently followed year after year [2].

Fiscal years often follow the business cycle of the organization. In the case of academic medicine, the fiscal year is most often identified as the academic year, beginning on July 1 and ending on June 30 of the following year. For the federal government, the fiscal year begins on October 1, ending on September 30 of the following year.

For one-time projects that are shorter than a year, the budget period is usually defined as the duration of the project.

An important principle to follow when constructing a budget and an important principle to consider when reviewing a budget is the accurate identification and timing of the revenues and expenses attached to the project, program, or organization. This "*matching principle*," the pairing of the expense to the revenue within the same time period, ensures that the budget reflects all of the revenues and expenses and reflects a true profit or loss or the true cost of the project [3].

An example of an extreme violation of the matching principle (and other GAAP principles) would be purposely omitting expected expenses, artificially lowering the budget, inflating a profit, or minimizing a loss.

Matching revenues and expenses to the correct budget period is a principle of "*accrual accounting*," a practice that recognizes a revenue or expense for a given activity in the period it was incurred, regardless of whether that revenue was actually collected or that expense was paid. "*Cash-based accounting*" or its variants recognize a revenue or expense when the cash is actually collected or the expense is paid regardless of when the activity attached to that revenue or expense occurred [3]. For example, a service is performed in year 20XX but the cash for that service is collected in 20XX + 1, the following year. Accrual-based accounting would recognize the revenue in 20XX, but cash-based accounting would recognize the revenue in 20XX + 1, the following year.

Medical group practices and medical schools often use a cash-based accounting method or one of its variants as the method to recognize both revenues and expenses [4].

Throughout the budget period, often quarterly if the budget period is a fiscal year, comparisons are made between actual performance and the budgeted performance. These comparisons result in "*budget variances*"—either a positive or negative indicator—highlighting the difference between what was budgeted versus what was actually realized, by revenue and expense category. An "actual versus budget" analysis appears in Fig. 22.2.

Finally, budget profits are identified as a positive number and in black ink (hence the term "in the black"), while budgeted deficits can be identified in red (hence the term "red ink"). A budget deficit is also often noted as a number bordered with parentheses, "($deficit)", or with a minus sign in front of the number, "-$deficit".

Reviewing Budgets

Academic faculty may be asked to construct and monitor their own budget, prospectively review other program budgets for approval, or be asked to evaluate an ongoing program's performance. Any of these reviews could occur in the education, research, or clinical program area.

Academic Medicine Department/Program
School of Medicine
University of State
July 1, 20XX - June 30, 20X+1

	Budget	**Actual**	**Variance**
Revenues	$ 135,000	$ 140,000	$ 5,000
Expenses			
Faculty Salaries	75,000	80,000	5,000
Staff Salaries	10,000	10,000	-
Fringe Benefits	25,500	27,000	1,500
Supplies & Expense	10,000	12,000	2,000
Other	5,000	4,000	(1,000)
Subtotal Expenses	$ 125,500	$ 133,000	$ 7,500
Total Profit (Loss)	$ 9,500	$ 7,000	$ (2,500)

Note: Variances can be positive and negative and care must be taken when evaluating variances on revenues and expenses. For example, a positive revenue variance would be "good" because the program has collected more revenues than budgeted. However a positive expense variance would be "bad" because the program has incurred more expenses than budgeted.

Fig. 22.2 Sample actual versus budget comparison and variance analysis

Monitoring Individual Budgets

After the faculty member constructs a budget that captures all identifiable revenues and expenses attached to the project or program, monitoring actual performance against the budgeted, expected performance is essential. Ensuring that the revenue and expenses actually realized are occurring at the level and pace that was expected is critical to a program's sustainability and success.

Revenues that underperform budgeted expectations or expenses that exceed budgeted expectations jeopardize a project, often attract unwanted organizational oversight, and sometimes result in the premature termination of a project or program. Monitoring the budget on a reasonable periodic basis through a variance analysis, as noted in Fig. 22.2, allows the faculty member to make adjustments to the budget as needed to ensure that program remains financially viable. For example, if revenues are underperforming, a faculty member might need to lower expenses to remain "in balance." Conversely, if revenues are exceeding expectations, the faculty member might be able to expand the project, that is, increase expenses, and still remain "in balance."

Evaluating Proposed Budgets

When prospectively evaluating a proposed budget, the faculty member can focus on at least two core questions, asking himself or herself the following:

Does the Budget Appear to Capture All of the Revenues and Expenses That Are Required to Do the Work?

\Omitting expense items such as personnel salaries or the benefits attached to personnel would be one glaring omission. Inadequately budgeted supplies, equipment, or travel expense items will damage the project, if not addressed in the prospective review, and will result in unfavorable budget variances once the program has started.

Is the Budget Reasonable?

There can be several tests for reasonableness when evaluating a budget, and these include:

- Can the work be realistically accomplished within the period identified?
- Is there enough faculty and staff effort dedicated to the project, and has this expense been fully addressed in the budget? In academic medicine, personnel salaries and benefits often consume 60–70 % of a budget unless large equipment purchases are part of the budget. Consequently, the reviewer can ask, does the faculty and staff effort identified match the work proposed? Table 22.1 describes in more detail how faculty and staff effort is measured.
- Are the underlying assumptions supporting the budget reasonable? For example, is space available for the program and has this cost been considered?

- If the budget is multiyear, are annual inflationary costs and performance increases for personnel included?
- If effort is expected to increase or decrease in the "out years" (years beyond the first year of the budgeted project), has this change in personnel cost been included?
- If equipment or other purchases are expected in the "out years," has this cost been included?
- Finally, do the revenues and expense budgets in the "out years" generally reflect the work that is proposed?

Evaluating Ongoing Performance

For evaluating another project or program's ongoing performance, the variance analysis as described in Fig. 22.2 is a useful tool. A review of the outcomes of the project or program and work performed will also likely accompany such a budget review, so the faculty member needs to be prepared to evaluate both "program and money" in such an instance.

Table 22.1 Measuring personnel effort

- Annualized full-time faculty or staff effort is considered to be 2080 h of work per year. When calculating an hourly rate of pay from an annualized salary, divide the annual salary by 2080. For example, a $50,000 annual salary will equate to a $24.04 hourly wage ($50,000/2080)
- Faculty and staff effort (time) is usually measured in "*full-time equivalents (FTE)*" identified as "percents of effort" where full-time effort equals 100 % or 1.0 FTE. Effort is usually evenly prorated; for example, half-time effort equals 50 % effort or 0.5 FTE. Any portion of faculty or staff effort can be identified in FTEs and can range as low as 5 % effort to 100 % effort, but never exceed 100 % effort
- For faculty and staff based in the Veteran's Administration (VA), effort is usually measured in eighths (1/8), where eight eighths (8/8) effort equals full time, 100 % effort or 1.0 FTE. Half-time work in the VA would be four eighths (4/8), equaling 50 % effort or 0.5 FTE. Any factor of one eighth can describe personnel effort in the VA system
- Federal grants measure faculty and staff effort in calendar months, where 12 months equals full time, 100 % effort, or 1.0 FTE. Half-time effort would be identified as 6 calendar months or 50 % effort and 0.5 FTE. Calendar months ranging from 1 to 12 can describe personnel effort in federal grant budget proposals

If the budgets extend over more than 1 year, the faculty reviewer should observe if the revenues and expenses are "trending" appropriately. Ongoing budgets for mature programs often extend over multiple years. When faced with multiyear budgets, an evaluation of the upward or downward trends in both the revenues and expenses provides the faculty reviewer a meaningful picture of the financial health of the program and the sustainability of the program. For example, are the program's revenues appropriately growing, one indication of a financially robust program? Are expenses growing too fast in relation to the revenues, a condition that might indicate future challenges? Conversely, are revenues declining, indicating a struggling program? These types of questions and their answers, arising from a "*trend analysis*," can assist the faculty member in his or her review and budget analysis.

A Federal Twist on Research and Other Program Budgets

If fundable research is part of the faculty member's academic world, he or she will encounter a federal twist or two that affect how a research project budget is constructed and reviewed.

Federally funded research budgets include both "*direct*" and "*indirect*" costs (also called "facility and administration" costs or "*F&A*"). Direct costs are generally defined as "salaries and benefits, consultant services, travel, materials, supplies and equipment and communication costs directly attributable to the award or activity" [5]. Indirect costs "represent the expenses of doing business that are not readily identified with a particular grant...but are necessary for the general operation of the organization and the conduct of activity it performs" [5]. These indirect costs of federally funded research are funded by an "indirect cost rate" and are calculated on the direct costs of the research grant budget. The indirect cost rate is established through an institutional negotiation with federal government officials, and this rate is then referenced in all grant budget submissions.

In the simplest of examples, if the negotiated indirect cost rate is 50 % and the direct costs of the grant total $100,000 annually, the indirect costs that accompany the grant will total $50,000 annually, for a total budget award of $150,000 annually.

Because of the indirect cost calculation, costs such as rent and other common institutional costs necessary for the conduct of federally funded research, which otherwise might appear in a proposed budget, do not appear in detail as part of the research project's direct costs. As such, reviewers need to ensure that proposed budgets only include the direct cost of the work and do not inadvertently itemize indirect costs—such as rent—as part of the proposed budget.

The federal government and other extramural funding agencies award grants throughout the calendar year, regardless of when the award falls within an institution's fiscal year. Consequently, grants can begin and end out of sync with the faculty member's fiscal year. In such instances, the faculty member needs to be cognizant of both the "grant year" and the institutional "fiscal year" when constructing and reviewing a budget.

Finally, as noted earlier and in Table 22.1, faculty and staff effort is measured in "calendar months" as opposed to "percent effort," another twist on budgeting for federal awards.

Conclusion

Reviewing a budget is a privilege the faculty member should welcome. Faculty members who are asked to review a budget are directly and indirectly being recognized for their expertise on a given topic, their experience with other projects, and their leadership in the academic setting.

Faculty will find more comfort and success when asked to review a budget by remembering some key principles and points such as:

- Sincerity, consistency, continuity, and good faith
- Completeness
- Reasonableness
- Properly matched revenues and expenses
- Budget variances
- Budget trends

Regardless of the venue or program area, consistently returning to these basic principles and conventions will help to ensure an

Words to the Wise
- Line graphs, pie charts, and other visuals are effective tools to describe budget performance.
- Budgets are often accompanied by comments, and sometimes these comments can be more revealing than the budget itself. For example, a comment about negative trends or other forecasts might offset an otherwise positive budget picture.
- Attention to detail is important when building a budget. Columns that are mislabeled, periods that are misidentified, and budget numbers that simply do not add up cast suspicion on the entire product or project.
- The budget message gets lost in too much explanation. Keep budgets simple, concise, and accurate for maximum effectiveness.
- Success for department heads, program leaders, researchers, and other faculty with budget responsibility lies in clearly understanding the components of the budget.

Ask Your Mentor or Colleagues
- What is the impact on the budget and on the project when no allowance for inflationary increases is calculated after the initial year of the project?
- Is a profit allowed in a federal grant budget?
- How does the indirect (F&A) calculation affect a project's budget?
- Is there ever an instance when revenues will exactly match the expenses?

informed faculty peer review of a proposed or ongoing budget.

References

1. Generally Accepted Accounting Principles; available at http://en.wikipedia.org/wiki/Generally_accepted_accounting_principles.
2. Fiscal Year; available at http://www.investorwords.com/1984/fiscal_year.html.
3. Welsch G, Zlatkovich C, Harrison W, et al. Intermediate accounting. 5th ed. Homewood, IL: Irwin; 1979.
4. Ross A, Williams S, Schafer E. Ambulatory care management. 2nd ed. Albany, NY: Delmar; 1991.
5. Indirect Cost Overview; available at http://www2.ed.gov/about/offices/list/ocfo/intro.html.

How to Engage in Departmental Strategic Planning

Robert C. Robbins, Diana Carmichael, and David O'Brien

Departments are the fundamental academic units of any university. As the university and individual departments evolve, it is imperative that a clear strategic vision and roadmap for individual departments be developed and frequently monitored. Departmental strategic plans provide the necessary framework to realize the higher-level institutional strategic visions with the current and potential activities of the department and its individual faculty. At its most basic level, it is through the actions of individual faculty that the missions of the institution are executed. Ideally, a strategic planning process should be completed in concert with changes in departmental leadership (both new appointments and renewals). Departmental strategic planning should be individualized reflections of the overall goals of the school and university and the specific strategic visions of the department and its faculty. Medical school clinical department plans must also reflect the

R.C. Robbins, M.D. (✉)
Texas Medical Center, 2450 Holcombe Boulevard, Suite One, Houston, TX, USA
e-mail: RCR@texasmedicalcenter.org

© Springer International Publishing Switzerland 2016   319
L.W. Roberts (ed.), *The Associate Professor Guidebook*,
DOI 10.1007/978-3-319-28001-1_23

strategic goals of their medical center partners. A department's strategic plan must address each of its core missions (education, research, and service/clinical care) in addition to other traditional areas of leadership and governance, faculty development, and resource management. Strategic planning is a leadership function, and, as such, it is absolutely necessary for the strategic planning process to be actively led by the department chair to ensure its success. However, it is also a community process and must involve all members of the department as well as other important partners and stakeholders outside the department. The use of professional strategic planners from within and outside the school will help to facilitate, bring order to the strategic planning process, and ensure an efficient and efficacious process. A comprehensive departmental strategic planning process will generally take approximately 6–9 months, and the majority of the work should be performed by a steering committee comprised of a small group of departmental members that will need to meet at least monthly. Once the plan has been developed, it should be presented to the entire department and other stakeholders prior to finalization.

Leadership

Academic departments function as small businesses led by department chairs who basically serve as de facto chief executive officers. The chairman's role in strategic planning is to unite and lead the faculty with a shared and compelling vision and oversee the tactical work required to execute the plan and achieve that vision. Although the department chair often has a clear vision for the department, a strategic planning process performed effectively will empower the faculty and staff to help shape the vision through specific goals and strategies to achieve the vision. Once completed, a strong departmental chair will delegate responsibility for many strategies to other faculty and staff leaders. The plan also should include metrics of success that can be utilized by the chairman to measure progress as the plan is executed.

Strategic Plan Components: Mission Areas

Clinical Programs

Strategic programmatic development is an important part of any strategic plan for clinical departments. The department must complete a comprehensive market and competitor analysis to fully understand unmet needs and opportunities for market share growth. These discussions should be done in conjunction with hospital partners, and ideally the clinical programs identified as strategic opportunities for growth will be well aligned with the department's research programs. The clinical section of a departmental strategic plan should include the following key components: (1) detailed marketing plans for targeted clinical programs using print, radio, television, web, and social media; (2) quality benchmark objectives should be developed in addition to clinical efficiency goals (both can be used in marketing plans and contract negotiations); and (3) clinical outreach strategies should be developed to maximize clinical referrals of profitable tertiary and quaternary cases.

Research Programs

The development of a detailed research program to discover new knowledge is central to any academic department's strategic plan. Opportunities in basic science, translational research, and clinical research should be considered. The research strategic planning deliberations should take into account current and potential research collaborators, current departmental strengths, and changing areas of investigation. Innovation and solutions to large problems will likely require interdisciplinary teams composed of investigators from other departments, schools within the university, other institutions, and corporate partners. Philanthropic funding for those targeted research programs identified for future growth as well as intramural funding from the dean's office or university institutes can provide the resources to begin new programs and permit longer term funding through grants and development of endowments.

Education Programs

Strategic teaching objectives are important for any academic department. Programs ranging from high school, undergraduate, graduate, postdoctoral, fellowship, continuing professional, to community educational programs should be considered in the department's strategic planning process. Curriculum changes should be carefully considered, and new educational programs should have clear goals, including funding sources. Simulation will continue to be an important part of any clinical educational program, especially for technically focused disciplines.

Strategic Plan Components: Resource Areas

Faculty

The recruitment, retention, and development of outstanding departmental faculty will be important to the success of the department, and plans for how to continuously help the departmental members evolve professionally should be a product of the strategic planning process. The mission-based strategies of the plan should capitalize on the strengths of the department's existing faculty and provide a clear roadmap for the recruitment of the future faculty needed to achieve the department's vision.

Finances

The strategic planning process should include a complete and transparent evaluation and discussion of departmental finances. A well-crafted plan for financial sustainability will be essential for the department to continue to grow and achieve academic success. Moreover, departments that have poor financial performance will create a stressful environment that will lead to underperformance and heavy scrutiny and potential micromanagement by the dean's office. Careful budgetary control and fiscal responsibility are important to maintain the department's healthy balance sheets. The strategic planning process should also include discussions about departmental compensation plans and investment. Development of strategies to increase clinical, teaching, research, and philanthropic funds should be aligned with targeted programmatic development. Clinical departments should include hospital administrative leadership in their planning process for programmatic development. Additionally, funds flow principles should be developed to include hospital medical direction funding and strategic programmatic investment. Strategic plans will invariably entail the need for targeted strategic investments. The vision and strategies included in the plan should be strong enough to make the case for investment by institutional leaders and donors.

Space

A comprehensive environmental resource analysis should be central to any academic departmental strategic plan. Academic office space, research laboratory, and clinical and educational spaces, including simulation space, should be considered during the strategic planning process. Creating plans for expansion of departmental space should be aligned with targeted programmatic development. As digital data become more expansive and important for clinical, educational, research, and administrative programs, the strategic plan must include provisions for adequate information, technical and bioinformatics space, and infrastructure support.

Staff

The recruitment, retention, and development of outstanding departmental staff will be important to the success of the department, and plans for how to continuously help the departmental members evolve professionally should be a product of the strategic planning process.

Organization

The strategic planning process should begin and end with a departmental organizational chart. Academic organizations are slow to change, and a current organizational chart provides an important reference point for where the department has been. But organizations are also a means to an end and, as such, should be carefully considered in the light of the department's vision, goals, and strategies. If necessary, a strategic plan should include a chart of the departmental organization that best reflects what the department hopes to be.

The departmental executive leadership team generally consists of division chiefs, a director of finance and administration, or business manager and vice chairs for academic affairs, research, and education. Each of these roles should be clearly delineated on the department's proposed organizational chart in the strategic plan.

Strategic Planning Methods

There should be a rigorous methodology to the strategic planning process, and this process should be facilitated by a strategy professional (Fig. 23.1). The department chair should assemble a diverse planning team, or strategic planning steering committee, that represents the various constituencies of the department. The orderly planning process should always begin with qualitative and quantitative assessments to establish where the department currently is and how it has gotten there over the past 3–5 years. The qualitative assessment should involve confidential interviews with key stakeholders within the department and the parent institution to gather input on current views of the department, important future opportunities, and the hope and dreams for the department. The quantitative assessment should include a thorough analysis of the key internal and external trends in each of the department's tripartite mission areas of research, patient care, and education.

In some instances, it may also be worthwhile to reach outside the institution in this assessment phase. Confidential interviews with selected thought leaders in the discipline can provide

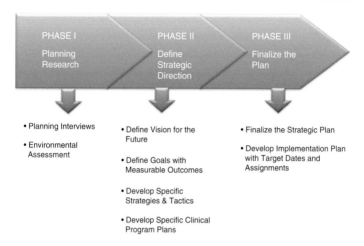

Fig. 23.1 The strategic planning process utilizes a three-phased approach with specific tasks assigned to each phase. The conclusions drawn from each phase established the foundation of planning for each of the subsequent phases. *Source*: AMC Strategies, LLC

valuable insights into key global treads that could inform on a department's strategic options. Collecting benchmark measures from peer departments can also be helpful in placing the department within an objective external context.

Based on the findings of each of these activities, the next phase of the planning process involves creating a mission statement and capturing a vision statement for the department. The mission statement should be a concise statement of purpose, reflecting the overarching reason why the members of the department perform their jobs. The vision of the department should capture the moon shot or comprehensive goal that the department aspires to achieve and should differentiate the department from the thousands of peer departments that exist globally. These two seemingly simple exercises are critical to the success of the strategic plan because these statements will guide every subsequent objective developed in the planning process. There will be healthy debate and meticulous attention to every word in each of these simple yet elegant statements. The group should be deliberate with this initial process and patiently work toward group consensus since these statements will not only guide the planning process but will also serve as the centerpiece of the marketing and communication of the department's strategic plan for the future. To avoid excessive wordsmithing by committee, it is often helpful to develop initial "working" versions of mission and vision statements and then revisit and refine them periodically throughout the process.

With a clear understanding of its environment and affirmations of its mission and vision, the department's strategic planning team can then move forward to develop a comprehensive set of goals and the tactics to achieve these goals over the next 5–10 years. A critical component of the plan is to embed metrics that can be used to monitor progress and measure success as the plan is implemented. A detailed analysis and resource plan must be completed, including estimates of the personnel (faculty and staff), financial, space, and political assets required to implement the plan, and their sources of support.

The plan should be presented in a slide deck format to the entire department and key stakeholders and then converted to a narrative that can be used as communication document for all the stakeholders and for fund-raising activities.

The execution of the strategic plan is obviously critical and will require focus and discipline by the leadership. Using metrics to assess the progress of achieving each goal is valuable, and the use of a timeline and dashboards to follow the progress on a quarterly basis is advisable.

Conclusion

Strategic planning is essential for the growth, evolution, and improvement of any successful academic department. This process should be performed with any changes in departmental leadership and at least every 5 years to ensure that the faculty and staff stay engaged and focused on the department's vision, commonly agreed-upon departmental goals, and the strategies to achieve the vision. The strategic plan should be comprehensive, have clear performance metrics, and should be used as documents for communicating the vision and goals of the department. It is important that the departmental strategic plan serves as a living document and be monitored and evaluated on at least an annual basis for refinement and to address any new trends or changes in the environment.

Words to the Wise
- Departmental strategic plans provide the framework to realize the higher-level institutional strategic visions with the current and potential activities of the department and its individual faculty.
- The strategic planning process should begin and end with a departmental organizational chart.
- The strategic planning process is best led by the department chair to ensure its success but is also a community process that must involve all members of the department as well as other important partners and stakeholders outside the department.

Ask Your Mentor or Colleagues
- What has been your experience with strategic planning?
- How do you recommend that I become involved in the process?

Index

© Springer International Publishing Switzerland 2016

L.W. Roberts (ed.), *The Associate Professor Guidebook*,

DOI 10.1007/978-3-319-28001-1

Printed in the United States
By Bookmasters